LIVE
LONGER
BETTER

LIVE LONGER BETTER

DR. ANDERSON'S COMPLETE
ANTIAGING HEALTH PROGRAM

JAMES W. ANDERSON, M.D. AND
MAURY M. BREECHER, M.P.H., PH.D.

PREFACE BY JEFFREY BLUMBERG, PH.D.

CARROLL & GRAF PUBLISHERS, INC.
NEW YORK

First published in hardcover in 1996 as *Dr. Anderson's Antioxidant, Antiaging Health Program*

Copyright © 1996 by James W. Anderson and Maury M. Breecher

Preface copyright © 1996 by Jeffrey Blumberg

Carroll & Graf Publishers, Inc.
19 W. 21st Street
New York, NY 10010

ISBN: 0-7867-0472-1

CIP Data for this edition is available.

Manufactured in the United States of America.

I dedicate this book to my family: Gay, Kathy, Steve, Tom, Allison, and Emily.

—James Anderson

I dedicate this book to my wife, Rebecca, and to my sons: Michael, who, as this book was being written, was taking his turn standing the Watch to preserve Peace as an Army paratrooper in Bosnia; Christopher, whose ambition and work ethic gratify my sense of fatherhood; and Martin, whose gentle caring and determination always warm me.

—Maury Breecher

ACKNOWLEDGMENTS

I (Anderson) appreciate the patience and support of my wife Gay and the assistance of Kathy Johnson and Belinda Smith.

I (Breecher) am grateful for the wonderful emotional support and editorial assistance of my wife, Rebecca Oxford, Ph.D.

We both appreciate the professionalism and encouragement of the entire Carroll & Graf team, especially publisher Kent Carroll and editor Jennifer Prior, as well as the scores of other individuals involved in creating, promoting, and otherwise marketing this book. We are also indebted to our agent, Jane Dystel.

CONTENTS

Preface: Dr. Jeffrey Blumberg, professor of Nutrition and
             chief, Antioxidants Research Laboratory,
             Tufts University, Boston   xi

Foreword: To the Reader   xv

Chapter 1: What Dr. Anderson's Antiaging Health Program
             Can Do for You   3

Chapter 2: Stay Young and Extend Your Productive Life Span   21

Chapter 3: Gain Protection Against Heart Disease and Stroke   34

Chapter 4: Protect Yourself Against Cancer   54

Chapter 5: Preserve Brain Function and Prevent
             Deterioration   73

Chapter 6: Prevent or Delay the Onset of Aging Skin,
             Arthritis, Diabetes, and Eye Diseases   87

Chapter 7: The Joys of Soy: Reduced Risks for Heart Disease,
             Cancer, and Osteoporosis   107

Chapter 8: Your Antioxidant Food and Supplement Program   123

Chapter 9: Wonderful Antioxidant, Antiaging Recipes   144

Chapter 10: Walk for the Health of It: Reduce Risks of
             Debilitating Disease   173

Chapter 11: Healthy Shopping, Cooking, and Eating Out   184

Chapter 12: Getting Started and Keeping Going   193

Chapter 13: Melatonin Update   200

Chapter 14: Putting Your Antioxidant, Antiaging Plan
             Together   212

x

Appendix A: *Antioxidant and Phytochemical Advisory*   219

Appendix B: *Table B*   226

Notes   229

Glossary   245

Index   257

PREFACE

It is now accepted that nutrition has a role in promoting optimal health and reducing the risk of chronic disease. This acceptance represents a paradigm shift—a dramatic transformation in the thinking of nutritionists and physicians that has evolved over the past twenty years. This change in thinking began with the acceptance of original research documenting that diets high in fat and low in fiber contribute significantly to the development of atherosclerosis, cancer, and other chronic diseases.

Within the last few years, an exciting new aspect of nutrition's ability to prolong healthy life spans has been discovered. Basic research and human studies have demonstrated the power of micronutrients—vitamins and minerals—to affect health beyond simply preventing or remedying deficiency diseases such as scurvy, beriberi, and pellagra. Realize that it was only during the first half of the twentieth century that vitamins and the amounts needed to prevent deficiencies resulting in those diseases were discovered. Those *preventive* intakes, quantified as the recommended dietary allowances (RDAs), have never been set in stone *because it has always been recognized that nutrition science is in a state of constant evolution.*

Now we have entered a new era of nutrition. The role of dietary factors, particularly the antioxidants, in the prevention of the major chronic diseases has been the focus of an ever-increasing body of scientific investigation. Compelling research studies have accumulated, particularly over the past five years, that demonstrate with remarkable consistency the benefits of antioxidants, such as beta-carotene and vitamins C and E. The evidence shows that these antioxidants enhance the functioning of certain organs and processes vital to the health and life of the body. The research has also shown that antioxidants work to counter the adverse impact of environmental toxicants such as smog and cigarette smoke and that they delay or prevent the onset of some of the most prevalent degenerative conditions that can afflict the human body.

For instance, many scientific studies have examined the relationship between micronutrients and cancer. With only a few exceptions, these studies have consistently identified a protective effect from generous intakes of the antioxidant vitamins C, E, and beta-carotene. High dietary and supplemental intakes of these antioxidant vitamins have also been associated with a lower incidence of cataracts, diabetes, heart disease, and infections. Vitamin D has been established as a critical nutrient in preventing age-related bone loss and osteoporosis. Data now suggest that increased consumption of several B vitamins, particularly folic acid, vitamin B_6 and vitamin B_{12}, can diminish circulating levels of homocysteine. This is a natural amino acid toxic to blood vessels and nerve cells that has been independently linked to coronary heart disease, stroke, and several neuropsychiatric disorders.

We are now beginning to appreciate that localized deficiencies of vitamins—even in the presence of what seemed to be adequate blood levels—are associated with pathological events. For example, inadequate levels of folic acid in the cervix are associated with cervical cancer, low amounts of vitamin E in the breast with fibrocystic breast disease, gastrointestinal deficiencies of vitamin C with gastric atrophy, and insufficient levels of beta-carotene in the mouth with precancerous lesions. Evaluations of the entire spectrum of available scientific evidence—from cell biology, animal studies, clinical trials, and epidemiological surveys—have earned the applause and approval of medical doctors and other clinicians. Improving nutritional status, in a rational fashion via changes in diet and supplementation, has proven both safe and inexpensive.

Media coverage of this exciting progress in nutritional research has attracted the attention of the general public. Today millions of people want to protect themselves and their families by applying the new knowledge. Ensuring appropriate intakes of protective nutrients, along with other healthy practices such as maintaining ideal body weight, stopping smoking, practicing safe sex, wearing seat belts, and exercising, joins the list of proactive, positive health behaviors that promote successful aging.

Abundant evidence indicates that a health care system that has the goal of promoting health and preventing illness will cost less than the present system, which basically operates to respond to the presence of illness with expensive diagnostic and therapeutic interventions. Consensus reports such as those from the U.S. surgeon general and National Research Council clearly support the notion of preventive nutrition.

Dr. Walter Bortz of Stanford University has declared that "we live too short and die too long." Life doesn't have to be like that. We can now begin to add years to our lives—and delay or even prevent the onset of certain chronic diseases—by applying what research has learned about our body's need for antioxidants and phytochemicals. The most important choices people can make to influence their long-term health prospects are in the area of nutrition.

These choices include knowledgeable selections of food and supplements. Foods should be chosen for their levels of nutrient enrichment, fortification, and for their antioxidant and phytochemical content. Supplements should be taken only if benefits have been well documented. This book can help people make these choices.

Jeffrey Blumberg, Ph.D., F.A.C.N.
Professor of Nutrition and Chief,
Antioxidants Research Laboratory
Tufts University, Boston

FOREWORD: TO THE READER

You have read about "the melatonin miracle," heard arguments about the benefits or lack of benefits of beta-carotene, seen *The Joys of Soy* on CNN. Your friends may be into heavy exercise and popping capsules containing substances called antioxidants and phytochemicals.

You want to add eight to twenty years to your life and protect yourself from debilitating diseases, but you are confused about how to accomplish these goals. You don't know what antioxidants and phytochemicals to take or in what quantity. You are also confused about what seems to be constantly changing exercise recommendations.

This book will eliminate the confusion. *Dr. Anderson's Antioxidant, Antiaging Health Program* clearly explains (in Chapters 1 and 2) what antioxidants are and what their role in the antiaging process is. In Chapter 3 and 4, you will discover how antioxidants and substances called phytochemicals protect you against heart disease and cancer. In a section in Chapter 4 entitled "The Great Vitamin Scares of 1994 and 1996," you will come to better understand controversies revolving about one of the those antioxidants, beta-carotene. In other chapters you will discover how antioxidants, especially vitamins C and E, work to protect your brain and delay or prevent skin aging, arthritis, diabetes, and eye diseases. In Chapter 13 you will learn about melatonin and how it helps sleep deprived individuals get a good night's sleep.

Before sending you on these explorations, may we ask you some questions?

To add eight to twenty healthy years to your life would you:

- commit an hour a day?
- spend $25 per week?

We have good news. You can lengthen your life span and enhance your health by investing *only thirty minutes per day and spending less than $10 per week.*

This practical book tells you:

1. what foods contain antiaging nutrients;
2. how much and which vitamin/mineral supplements you need;
3. the latest information on nutritional breakthroughs involving substances called phytochemicals, Pycnogenol, and soy proteins;
4. how to increase your chances of avoiding Alzheimer's disease, cancer, and heart attacks;
5. what types and amounts of exercise to do.

Read this book with pen in hand to make a shopping list—one that will cost you less than $10 a week for the life-saving nutrients. These nutrients, plus thirty minutes per day, will enhance your vitality and help you live longer.

Here's to your good health.

LIVE
LONGER
BETTER

1

What Dr. Anderson's Antiaging Health Program Can Do for You

You want to live longer, be healthier, and feel more energetic. That's why you are looking at this book. We can help you achieve these goals.

Do you spend an hour a day watching television? You need to spend half that amount of time *on your health* each day (a bit more for people with certain risk factors or a chronic disease). Your reward will be improved health, increased vitality, and a slowing of the aging process.

With the knowledge contained in this book, this small commitment of time and money can help you enjoy a *longer, healthier, more energetic, more productive life.* In a systematic, easy-to-understand manner, this book provides the skills and knowledge you need to obtain these benefits. As a bonus, if you need to lose weight, the eating plan in Chapter 8 will enable you to permanently lose—at a safe, nonstressful rate—those unhealthy, fatigue-producing extra pounds.

4

ANTIOXIDANTS, FREE RADICALS, AND PHYTOCHEMICALS

Antioxidants and other phytochemicals (phyto = plant) are Mother Nature's protection from assaults by *free radicals*. Free radicals are *not* escaped terrorists. The term refers to unstable oxygen molecules that punch holes into our body's cellular walls, damaging DNA, the genetic material within. As this damage accumulates, our bodies become rusty, like an old car. A rust bucket of a car is likely to break down. A body damaged by free radicals has a reduced capability to combat aging, cancer, hardening of the arteries, and other degenerative changes.

FRANK & ERNEST

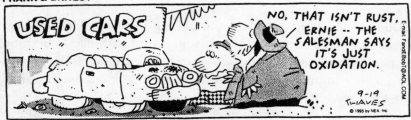

Reprinted by permission of Newspaper Enterprise Association, Inc.

The way to get protection from these tiny destroyers is to avoid rust inducers—cigarette smoke, environmental pollutants, and irradiation—and get generous amounts of the phytochemicals and antioxidants from one's daily diet and from supplements. Our early hunter-gatherer ancestors did not have cigarettes or modern-day environment pollutants to harm them. The sun was their only source of irradiation. Besides having fewer toxic environmental stressors, their regular eating pattern included great amounts of vegetables, fruits, nuts, and legumes, so they often had very high antioxidant and phytochemical intakes. Rather than dying from attacks from within (free radicals), our primitive ancestors died from attacks from without—wild animals, warring tribes, and diseases that struck during times of famine when their natural immune defenses had been weakened.

How Antioxidants Work

Scientists believe that compounds like vitamin E, known as antioxidants, may help thwart many common diseases by taming harmful molecules known as free radicals.

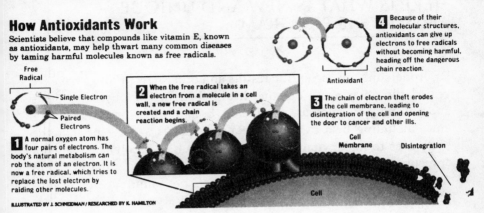

Free Radical
— Single Electron
— Paired Electrons

1 A normal oxygen atom has four pairs of electrons. The body's natural metabolism can rob the atom of an electron. It is now a free radical, which tries to replace the lost electron by raiding other molecules.

2 When the free radical takes an electron from a molecule in a cell wall, a new free radical is created and a chain reaction begins.

3 The chain of electron theft erodes the cell membrane, leading to disintegration of the cell and opening the door to cancer and other ills.

4 Because of their molecular structures, antioxidants can give up electrons to free radicals without becoming harmful, heading off the dangerous chain reaction.

Antioxidant

Cell Membrane   Disintegration

Cell

ILLUSTRATED BY J. SCHNEIDMAN / RESEARCHED BY K. HAMILTON

It has only been relatively recently that scientists have discovered the immunity-boosting, antiaging, health-promoting effects of antioxidants and phytochemicals. Today excellent medical and nutritional research provides evidence that these substances can offer protection against premature aging and delay or even reverse some chronic diseases. Although hundreds of newspaper and magazine articles have been written on phytochemicals and even more have been written on antioxidants, most consumers are still confused about what these substances are, how they protect us, and how to ensure proper nutrition by using them. That's because single articles, no matter how well written, cannot provide all the information needed to make use of the new research. This book provides this information in an easy-to-understand-and-use, comprehensive health plan to increase longevity and promote vitality. Our program does not ask you to move to some remote island and return to a primitive lifestyle. Rather, we outline how you can fight the internal demons in the comfort of your own home, car, and workplace.

HERE IS WHAT IS NEW AND UNIQUE ABOUT THIS PROGRAM

Dr. Anderson's own scientific results and other new findings have revealed the amazing, protective health benefits of phytochemicals and antioxidants such as vitamins C, E, and other important nutrients, including beta-carotene. Beta-carotene is a nutrient that the body uses to make vitamin A. (That's why beta-carotene is called a "precursor" of vitamin A.) In fact, beta-carotene is safer than vitamin A. Too much vitamin A causes side effects not found when one simply takes beta-carotene and allows the body to make as much vitamin A as it needs.

Dr. Anderson's antiaging program is the first book to rigorously examine and explain in clear language how antioxidants and phytochemicals work together to resist the ravages of aging and improve your overall health. We explain groundbreaking studies that provide you with knowledge that can be used right away to dramatically improve your health and extend your life.

The new studies and Dr. Anderson's own research and experience with patients have been used to develop a total health program that has two attributes:

1. It really works.
2. You can easily incorporate the program into your own life.

There's good news from the world of exercise research also. No longer is it necessary to exhaust yourself to win health benefits from exercise. In fact, those who do high-intensity exercise generate huge numbers of dangerous free radicals. We will tell you more about the exercise connection in Chapter 10. Right now you need to learn more about those hazardous substances known as free radicals.

THE FREE RADICAL STORY

Oxygen is the breath of life; without it, we die. Humans, like all oxygen-dependent life on the planet Earth, have made a Faustian bargain. The very air we breathe contains oxygen necessary to life. Oxygen, though, can combine with other elements within the body, releasing energy in the life-giving natural process called oxidation. The process of oxidation has its dark side, however. Over time, the process—the free radical chain of oxidation—causes whatever it touches to rust or turn rancid.

Almost everything on earth is gradually oxidizing. It's part of the cycle of life. As Dr. William A. Pryor, a leading antioxidant researcher at Louisiana State University, points out, "Almost everything is gradually oxidized by oxygen: Fats turn rancid, rubber loses elasticity, paper turns brown, and even iron gradually rusts in air. Thus it is not surprising that the cells of all plants and animals show a continuous level of oxidative damage."[1]

Take a bite out of an apple and expose it to the air for a few minutes. The exposed flesh of the apple soon turns brown. That's oxidation at work. Oxidation provides needed energy for life, yet within our bodies the process is a two-edged sword. Unfortunately, a small number of the oxygen molecules we breathe is converted within our bodies to unstable free radicals. Free radical-caused oxidation produces premature aging and sets us up for serious illness, including cancer and heart disease. Natalie Angier, science reporter for *The New York Times,* calls the damage caused by free radicals "the price we pay for breathing."[2]

Researchers now understand how free radicals are formed. Free radical oxygen molecules are unstable because each lacks an electron. An oxygen atom normally has a nucleus with paired electrons orbiting around it. Free radicals have an unpaired electron. It is the nature of these renegade molecules to seek out and steal an electron from any cell membrane or structure it strikes. The result is a cascading chain reaction of free radicals causing damage throughout the cells of our bodies. The most-studied free radical chain reaction in living systems is lipid peroxidation. The term "lipid" refers to any fat-soluble substance, animal or vegetable. "Peroxidation" refers to the formation of peroxide molecules, molecules that contain the greatest proportion of oxygen atoms.

Ninety-eight percent of the oxygen we breathe is used by tiny powerhouses within our cells called mitochondria, which convert sugar, fats, and oxygen into the energy we need to live. In this energy-producing process, a small percentage of the leftover oxygen loses electrons, creating those destructive demons within called free radicals. These free radicals burn holes in our cellular membranes. Calcium penetrates our cells through these holes. This calcium overload can lead to cell death, which, in turn, weakens tissues and organs. As this damage accumulates, our bodies become, like the junky old car mentioned earlier, "rusty" and less able to fight off cancer, hardening of the arteries, premature aging, and other bodily disorders.

Every nine seconds each of the 63 trillion cells in our bodies takes an oxidative "hit." Our bodies accumulate 630 quadrillion damaging blows per day. Each strike by a free radical leaves a scar that can lead to further damage and even death of the cell. Each of those 63 trillion cells contains 23 pairs of thin strands of the genetic material known as DNA. Of the 630 quadrillion blows, each cell takes about 10,000 and each DNA strand gets hit approximately 5,000 times per day. Each strand has an identical twin that backs up our genetic code. The free radical bombardment causes a typical human cell to undergo thousands of changes or mutations daily. Although each mutation can turn cancerous, it occurs rather rarely because carcinogenic mutations must occur on both strands of DNA at or about the same time. Although both strands of DNA are under bombardment by free radicals, damage on one or the other strands is usually repaired before the cancer process can begin. Yet, when these cellular repair mechanisms lack the right amounts of antioxidants and phytochemicals, they become overwhelmed, and the risks for cancer and premature aging increase.

WHAT ARE ANTIOXIDANTS AND PHYTOCHEMICALS, AND HOW DO THEY PROTECT US?

One key to stopping premature aging and preventing many degenerative diseases is for the body to be able to repair the damage that does occur. The other key is to protect the body's tissue cells from the free radicals before they cause mutations. Antioxidants are substances with free-radical chain-reaction-breaking properties. They include any substance that significantly delays, inhibits, or prevents oxidation caused by free radicals. Phytochemicals are literally chemicals that come from plants. These plant chemicals fight many diseases. Many phytochemicals are antioxidants, but they also have other properties, such as stimulating plant growth, and providing color to plants and flavor to vegetables. In humans, phytochemicals enhance the body's own healing powers. More than 60,000 of these plant chemicals have been discovered. From observation, healers know that many have specific healing properties, yet sorting out which ones are responsible for what healing properties will take scientists years of research.

Each cell produces its own antioxidants, but the ability to produce them decreases as we age. That's why a diet high in antioxidant- and phytochemical-rich fruits and vegetables supplemented with additional vitamins and minerals is important. These substances contribute significantly to our defenses against oxidative damage and thus protect against premature aging and disease. No matter whether these protectors are produced by the body or ingested through food or supplements, they work to protect us by:

1. preventing the formation of some free radicals;
2. intercepting and absorbing free radicals after those destructive devils are formed;
3. helping cells repair oxidative damage;

4. eliminating damaged molecules;
5. minimizing the number of mutations.[3]

In other words, antioxidants act as vital heroes, shielding the cell's DNA from free radical bombardment and protecting the interior of the cell by absorbing free radicals and damaged molecules. This protection reduces the number of mutations resulting from the injury-causing molecular outlaws.[4]

Phytochemicals work with antioxidants by aiding the cell's own reparative functions. Phytochemicals also protect us from toxic chemicals in the environment by deactivating them. Exactly how they do this is the subject of ongoing research.

FREE RADICALS CAN ALSO PROTECT US, BUT UNCONTROLLED, THEY WRECK US

We do know the details of how antioxidants work. They combat renegade free radicals. Ironically, not all free radicals are bad. White blood cells create free radicals to protect the body against invading bacteria and viruses. To kill these foreign invaders, white blood cells strip electrons from oxygen molecules. Most of the newly created free radicals do what they are supposed to do—smash into and obliterate the foreign invaders. Unfortunately, free radicals don't attack just bacteria and viruses. As we have seen, outlaw free radicals also attack healthy cells, cellular membranes, and even DNA (the genetic material within the cell's nucleus). The body tries to balance the excess production of free radicals by using antioxidants and special phytochemical enzymes as free radical scavengers.

WHAT WILL THE ANTIOXIDANT PROGRAM DO FOR ME?

Knowledge about antioxidants is mushrooming, exploding, rocketing through the stratosphere, or as Dr. Anderson's teenage nephew says, "awesome." We tell you about the very latest research, but you will need to continue to watch your daily newspaper or weekly news magazine for information discovered or published after early 1996. Current research indicates than an antioxidant- and phytochemical-rich diet will reduce your risk for these health problems:

- *heart attack, stroke,* and *hardening of the arteries* by lowering blood cholesterol levels and protecting low-density lipoproteins (LDLs), the "bad guy" cholesterol, from becoming oxidized and accumulating as plaque in the blood vessels;
- *cancer* by inactivating toxic chemicals and radiation, preventing oxidation of DNA, blocking initiation of cancer-prone cells, stopping conversion of precancerous cells to cancerous ones, and enhancing the immune system to fight tumorous cells;
- *aging* by slowing down the rusting process that affects all cells;
- *Alzheimer's disease* by preventing oxidative damage to brain cells and accumulation of damaged protein (amyloid) deposits;
- *diabetes* by slowing down oxidative damage to the beta cells on the pancreas, which manufacture insulin;
- *certain eye diseases* such as age-related macular degeneration (ARMD) and cataracts, which are the result of oxidative damage to the eyes;
- *arthritis,* which often results from an ineffective immune system;
- *osteoporosis,* which can be substantially slowed by intake of generous amounts of calcium and soy protein.

WHY CAN'T I JUST TAKE SUPPLEMENTS TO PROTECT MY HEALTH?

Supplements are important, and we will tell you which ones and how much. However, because medical science doesn't yet know all there is to know about antioxidants and phytochemicals, supplements cannot contain all the protective nutrients that our bodies need. For example, you need to eat soy protein to get genistein and daidzein, important soy substances called isoflavones. Those soy chemicals lower blood cholesterol, protect against heart attack and stroke, reduce risks of breast and prostate cancers, slow the process of osteoporosis, and have other health benefits. You can't get all that from a supplement capsule. However, we do know the beneficial effects of some supplements, and those are the ones we recommend (see Chapter 8).

As mentioned before, the body makes some of its own antioxidants, but as we age, we partially lose this ability. That's why it is important to eat plenty of fruits and vegetables, natural sources of both antioxidants and phytochemicals. However, because of poor dietary choices, most people don't get enough of those protective substances. "Only 9 percent of Americans eat the recommended five servings of fruits and vegetables per day," says noted cancer researcher Dr. Bruce Ames.[5] The result: excess production of free radicals, which injure vital bodily structures.

Important studies provide evidence that regular intake of phytochemical- and antioxidant-rich foods, and a few antioxidant supplements, combats free radicals and strengthens our immune systems, thus also combating other disease processes. Eating properly and taking "insurance" doses of the supplemental nutrients recommended in Chapter 8 will reduce your risks of developing many of the infirmities associated with premature aging.

Although we don't have a special weight-loss section, if you are overweight you'll find that the antioxidant, antiaging food plan portion of this book—with its tasty, specially tailored menus and easy-to-cook recipes featuring phytochemical- and antioxidant-rich foods—will help you shed unhealthy excess weight. It makes sense that if you fill up with nutrient-dense, high-fiber, phytochemical- and antioxidant-rich foods—and cut your intake of fats as recommended—you will lose weight. That's a bonus for those who are overweight.

Now let's look at two people who achieved better health using the antioxidant, antiaging program.

SALLY'S SUCCESS STORY

Sally, a thirty-four-year-old office manager, came to see me (Dr. Anderson) because she had retained too much weight after having two children. At 5 feet, 6 inches she had weighed 130 pounds after college, when she was married. After having and nursing two children, her weight had ballooned to more than 160 pounds. She tried various diet plans, but although she lost some weight initially, she was unable to keep it off and regained more than she had lost. In addition to being overweight, she was concerned about her blood pressure and cholesterol levels. At the time of her examination, Sally weighed 165 pounds, had a blood pressure of 142/88, a serum cholesterol value of 247 mg per 100 ml, and a serum triglyceride level of 223 mg per 100 ml. We considered these values too high, so we started her on antioxidant supplements tailored to her needs, helped her identify antioxidant-rich foods that she liked, and instructed her on how to implement the rest of my antiaging health program, including how to exercise correctly so as not to create more free radicals.

Sally enthusiastically embarked on the program. She began keeping meticulous records of her food intake and exercise, she shopped for foods high in antioxidants, and she took her supplements as recommended twice daily. She spent forty-five minutes walking two miles daily. Without experiencing hunger or feelings of deprivation,

Sally lost 9 pounds of excess weight in the first month. When she came into the office, her blood pressure was 126/76 and her serum cholesterol value was 198 mg per 100 ml, reductions that pleased me.

Encouraged by this progress, Sally intensified her exercise program. She began spending twenty minutes per day working out to the beat of an exercise video, and she accelerated her walking speed to three miles in forty-five minutes. Her husband, Dick, was pleased because the whole family was now eating the antioxidant way, and he had lost 8 pounds. Both parents felt good about feeding their children a healthier diet. Sally continued to keep records of her food and exercise and lost 7 pounds in the second month of the antiaging health program.

Sally began sharing shopping and cooking tips with family members and friends. These activities put pressure on her to maintain her own success, and she did. By the end of six months she had achieved her weight goal of 135 pounds, and her blood pressure, serum cholesterol, and serum triglycerides were in the safe zones. Not only did Sally feel good about her own health, she also felt she was helping her family do healthy things. Now they were walking or bike-riding together, they ate nutritious meals, and they selected vegetables and fruits high in antioxidants for snacks. Even the children enjoyed the fresh vegetable juice that Sally or Dick made two or three times weekly. One year later, Sally is maintaining her ideal weight. Here is her scorecard:

TABLE 1.1   SALLY'S SCORECARD

MEASURE	INITIAL	1 MONTH	3 MONTHS	6 MONTHS	GOAL
Weight	165	156	144	135	≤143
Blood pressure	142/88	126/76	116/68	112/66	≤120/80
Cholesterol	247	198	189	193	≤200
Triglycerides	223	157	142	135	≤150
Exercise*	0	2	3	4	3

* Exercise is converted into estimated miles walked per day.

KENTUCKY BASKETBALL STAR SLAM-DUNKS BLOOD CHOLESTEROL

Bill was an All-American basketball player at the University of Kentucky and an All-Pro for several years during his National Basketball Association career. After retiring from professional basketball, he returned to Lexington, Kentucky, to manage an insurance agency. As time passed, Bill became rather sedentary and began to smoke several packs of cigarettes per day. Worried because he was nearing age fifty, a time of life when several members of his family had heart attacks or strokes, Bill came to see me.

When I saw Bill, he appeared to be in excellent health except for his weight. First appearances were deceiving: His blood cholesterol levels were a scary 317 mg/100 ml. (Healthy cholesterol levels are lower than 200 mg/100 ml.) His HDL (the "good guy" component of cholesterol) level was low, at 37 (see Bill's scorecard). Although an exercise stress test showed that Bill's heart was not yet injured, the high blood fat readings were setting the stage for later medical problems.

Bill had two choices: take pills for the rest of his life to lower his cholesterol, or participate in the antioxidant, antiaging health program. He didn't want to take pills all of his life and asked about his other option. I told Bill that if he wanted to live a long and healthy life he *must* stop smoking, take recommended amounts of supplemental antioxidant nutrients, and lose at least ten pounds. I assured him that if he followed my program he would add many healthy years to his life span.

Bill enthusiastically agreed to comply with these recommendations and pursued them with the same determination and intensity that he had used to captain the basketball team. He immediately stopped smoking and started walking one mile each evening with his wife, Connie. Both Bill and Connie met with a dietitian who explained how to use the food plan portion of my antiaging health program to incorporate phytochemical- and antioxidant-rich foods in their diets.

On my recommendation, Bill also started taking supplemental antioxidant vitamins. We were in the early stages of our antioxidant research, so I recommended what I considered to be the best regimen for his condition at that time: 16,000 IU (9.6 mg) of beta-carotene, 1,000 mg of vitamin C, and 400 IU of vitamin E. (Today I would have doubled his intake of vitamin E.)

Over the next year, Bill increased his walking to six or sometimes even ten miles per week, followed Dr. Anderson's antiaging food plan most of the time, and took the recommended doses of supplemental vitamins. The results were good. His weight and cholesterol levels dropped. His total blood lipids plummeted by 73 points, and his HDL ("good guy") cholesterol increased by 24 percent, into the normal range.

Bill and I still were not satisfied with his blood fat levels or his weight, so we intensified the program. He promised to follow the food plan better, increase his exercise, and lose even more weight. Over the next two years Bill became active in food shopping and even began to do some of the cooking. He is now very knowledgeable about the best phytochemical- and antioxidant-rich foods to eat and ways to cook them. (You can be, too. See Chapters 7, 8, 9, and 11.) Bill has also continued taking antioxidant supplements and has increased his walks to twelve to fifteen miles per week. These steps produced dramatic results. He lost another ten pounds. His total blood lipids, including LDL ("bad guy") cholesterol and HDL ("good guy") cholesterol, moved into very healthy ranges. In fact, when these new results arrived at my office, I thought that the laboratory must have made a mistake, so I asked Bill to return for another blood test. The second test confirmed the dramatic improvements.

Here is Bill's scorecard. He achieved these results without the use of cholesterol-lowering medicines.

TABLE 1.2   BILL'S SCORECARD

MEASURE	INITIAL	1 YEAR	3 YEARS	GOAL
Weight	242	239	229	≤231
Cholesterol	317	244	175	≤200
LDL ("bad guy") cholesterol	209	132	72	≤130
HDL ("good guy") cholesterol	37	54	60	≥45

TO SUM UP

• Sally, a thirty-four-year-old office manager, weighed too much and had high blood pressure and serum cholesterol and serum triglyceride levels that were unhealthy. With the proper food choices, increased exercise, and antioxidant supplements, she eliminated these unhealthy risk factors.

• Bill, a former University of Kentucky basketball superstar, had staggering levels of cholesterol in his blood before he enrolled in our program. Like Sally, by using the antioxidant program of diet, exercise, and antioxidant supplements he was successful in dramatically decreasing those high lipid levels. He not only decreased his LDL ("bad guy") cholesterol but also raised his HDL ("good guys"). His risk of heart attack is now well less than what it was.

• Much of the aging in our bodies relates to damage from toxic free radicals. These demons from within punch through the outer cell walls and injure the DNA within. The injuries can lead to cell death, cell dysfunction, or worse—transformation of the injured cells into cancerous ones (see Chapter 4).

• Antioxidants such as beta-carotene, vitamin C, and vitamin E protect cells from damage by free radicals. The antioxidants even repair damage to cell walls and to DNA.

• Phytochemicals (plant chemicals) protect us from toxic substances by inactivating them, preventing and repairing damage to cells.

• Soy isoflavones are a special type of phytochemical that have antioxidant and other protective properties that enable them to decrease blood cholesterol levels and protect us from heart disease, breast or prostate cancer, osteoporosis, and other diseases.

• Full benefits from Dr. Anderson's antiaging health program come from eating antioxidant- and phytochemical-rich vegetables and fruits *and* taking appropriate supplements. Supplement capsules alone can't provide full protection.

• This antioxidant, antiaging health program offers protection from premature aging; heart disease, stroke, and hardening of the arteries; cancer; Alzheimer's disease; arthritis; diabetes; osteoporosis; and certain eye diseases, such as macular degeneration and cataracts.

• The antioxidant, antiaging health program is a *comprehensive* plan that incorporates not only new nutritional research but also studies in the field of exercise physiology. The result is an antiaging health program consisting of three levels:

1. The first, a general protection level, is for people in good health without specific disease risk factors. This general protective level consists of suggested phytochemical- and antioxidant-rich foods, a diet in which one's fat intake is 30 percent or less, antioxidant vitamin and mineral supplements, easy walking and upper body exercises, and other healthwise behaviors.

2. To postpone or even prevent disease, the second level consists of a tailored, disease-prevention regimen. This part of the health program is for people with such risk factors as family histories of heart attack, stroke, blood clots before age fifty, or Alzheimer's disease. People at this level are advised to eat phytochemical- and antioxidant-rich foods and to restrict their fat intake to 25 percent or less total calories. They are also encouraged to take twice the amount of certain antioxidant vitamins and minerals, to walk a few miles more, and to do thirty minutes more per week of gentle upper body exercise.

3. The third level is designed to encourage disease reversal for people who are already sick. This level also emphasizes phytochemical- and antioxidant-rich foods; a reduced total fat calorie intake of 20 percent or less; various supplements, including fish oil capsules; and engaging in slightly more upper body exercises. It is

important for people at this level to *continue their regular medical care*. We aren't claiming that this program is a cure-all. That would be like the old-time medicine show snake oil salespeople. However, the antioxidant, antiaging health program, combined with proper medical care, is one's best bet to beat back and prevent disease and extend one's productive life span. That's why we say this program can help people achieve what for them is their own individual optimal health.

WHAT YOU CAN DO NOW

- Read this book, take notes, and go grocery and supplement shopping.
- Concentrate on Chapter 2 if you are keenly interested in increasing longevity.
- Concentrate on Chapter 3 if heart disease is a worry or if it occurs frequently and early in your family.
- Concentrate on Chapter 4 if you are especially concerned about cancer or if it has occurred frequently in your family.
- Concentrate on Chapter 5 if you need to know about Alzheimer's or Parkinson's diseases or if either or both of these conditions have occurred in your family.
- Concentrate on Chapter 6 if you are concerned about arthritis, diabetes, eye diseases, or skin problems.
- Concentrate on Chapter 7 if you want to learn about the exciting benefits of soy products.
- Concentrate on Chapter 8 for full details of the food portion of the program.
- Use Chapter 9 to obtain delicious antiaging recipes.
- Peruse Chapter 10, which explains that you don't have to kill yourself to get the health and longevity benefits of exercise. We tell you what types of low-intensity exercises are best.
- Read Chapter 11, which gives valuable advice about food shopping, cooking, and eating out.

- With Chapter 12, jump-start your motivation to get started on the antiaging program.
- Learn about the sleep-producing effects of melatonin in Chapter 13.
- Pull your entire antioxidant, antiaging program together with Chapter 14. It steps you through the process of starting, advancing to the second level, and sustaining the good health you will attain with the full program.

Once you begin this program, you'll feel more energetic and be able to enjoy a longer, healthier, more vibrant life. Remember, *eat for the health of it and walk as though your life depends on it. It does.*

2

STAY YOUNG AND EXTEND YOUR PRODUCTIVE LIFE SPAN

Meet Martin and Suzanne.[1] Martin, a successful lawyer, is sixty pounds overweight. A hard-driving workaholic all of his adult life, Martin has carried a secret fear for thirty-nine years. When Martin was twelve, his father, Morgan, died of a heart attack at age fifty-two. Martin recently celebrated his fifty-first birthday and fears that healthwise he is following in his father's footsteps. His doctor told him he had dangerously high blood cholesterol and triglyceride levels. Like his father, Martin has been married three times and has three sons from his first two marriages: Tom, twenty-nine, who is as much overweight as his dad; Sam, twenty-five, who is just now starting to put on excess weight; and Ronald, nineteen, the son from his second marriage. As a paratrooper in the U.S. Army, Ronald now enjoys peak physical fitness.

Martin wants to live long enough to see his sons marry, have children, and make him a grandfather. He longs to be a good health model for his sons and grandchildren. He began Dr. Anderson's health program in the fall of 1995. Although he still has a long way to go, he is losing weight and his blood cholesterol and triglyceride levels have dropped to safer levels.

Suzanne is a thirty-six-year-old hair stylist. Since the birth of her second child she has been thirty pounds overweight. In the past she often complained about her "uncontrollable sweet tooth." Then she developed Type II (adult-onset) diabetes about two years ago. Because her diabetes was controlled by glipizide (a pill that stimulates the pancreas to produce more insulin), she thought she wouldn't have to alter her poor eating habits. Foolishly, she refused to take any doctor or nutritionist's dietary advice. She admits that she was foolish and regrets those decisions now. Soon the pills failed to properly control her blood sugar levels. After she experienced extreme fatigue and night sweats, a blood test revealed that Suzanne had been having dangerously high blood sugar levels for several months. Her doctor put her on insulin and convinced her to use a blood sugar monitoring device at home. She had to take two shots of Humulin 70/30 insulin per day. Suzanne learned about Dr. Anderson's antiaging health program from the coauthor of this book, Dr. Breecher. Suzanne said she was finally ready to make changes in her life and eagerly agreed to begin both the food portion of Dr. Anderson's antiaging health program and the exercises described later in this book. She confided that her newfound enthusiasm was because she also had a secret fear: Her mother had died at age forty-two of acidosis, a side effect of undiagnosed diabetes; Suzanne feared that she, too, would die young.

Suzanne now has changed what she eats. She walks several miles each day and reports feeling more energetic. Although she still has to take insulin, the amount she takes has dropped by a third, and her fasting (before breakfast) blood sugar levels are down to about 140, good for a diabetic but still outside the 80–120 range that people without diabetes usually have after waking up.

Both Martin and Suzanne are doing much better now. Their chances of living significantly longer than their parents are good.

You may not share Martin or Suzanne's specific health problems, but you probably feel the need to do something to increase your odds for a long and healthy life span. It is normal to want to avoid the physical and mental deterioration associated with aging and escape diseases of the heart, lungs, and kidneys. In most people the ability of these organs to function optimally declines as they age. Many killer diseases, including cancer, coronary heart disease, and diabetes, are found with higher frequency in older people. As we age, we can fall prey to ailments that limit our enjoyment of life: fading vision, brittle bones, stiff joints, muscle weakness, and skin problems.

Cheer up! It is *not* inevitable that your body has to degenerate *just because you are getting older.* We have the right to live full, vital lives. The foods you eat, the phytochemical/antioxidant supplements you take, the exercise you do, and an upbeat attitude can positively affect your body's ability to prevent diseases and other ailments associated with premature aging.

In this chapter we discuss various theories of aging and explain how Dr. Anderson's program works to prolong healthy life spans. Prudent exercise, antioxidant-rich foods, and supplements of vitamin C, vitamin E, beta-carotene, and phytochemical supplements such as Pycnogenol are cornerstones of Dr. Anderson's antiaging treatment.[2] In later chapters we provide specific recommendations, depending on your health status and heredity, about phytochemical- and antioxidant-rich foods and provide advice about the substances you should take as supplements, the amount of low-intensity exercise you should do, and other healthful, life-extending measures.

THEORIES OF AGING

Aging is a complex process not yet totally understood by scientists.[3] Current theories of aging have been simplified into four possible mechanisms: immunologic, metabolic, genetic, and wear-and-tear free radical. Let's briefly look at the first three theories to better understand how antioxidants may help. The fourth theory, one currently popular with many researchers, is the wear-and-tear theory. That theory meshes extremely well with what researchers have found to be the antiaging properties of phytochemicals and antioxidants. Let's look at those theories one by one.

THE IMMUNOLOGIC THEORY

With advancing age, the human immune system undergoes progressive deterioration. Part of that decline relates to the shrinking of an organ known as the thymus. For years scientists have known that deficiencies in certain vitamins and other substances (vitamins A, C, and E, the B vitamin folic acid, the phytochemicals, and possibly the hormone melatonin) weaken the ability of the thymus to produce adequate numbers of T cells.

T cells act as scouts and soldiers to first identify and then kill foreign invaders such as bacteria, viruses, fungi, or parasites. When T cells aren't produced in sufficient numbers, we become prey to any number of debilitating infections. Responding to infections, our immune systems also generate free radicals. This can be beneficial in the short term but harmful in the long run.

However, new studies show that even modest amounts of antioxidant supplementation protect against nutritional deficiencies, help sop up excess free radicals, and thus strengthen the immune system.[4] Research has consistently shown that individuals who eat diets rich in antioxidants have reduced rates of infectious disease. Hundreds of other scientific studies provide evidence that proper antioxidant nutrition also acts to enhance the body's ability to repair itself. That's why it is imperative that we improve our diets with antioxidants and develop healthy lifestyle habits (see Table 8.1 in Chapter 8).

THE METABOLIC THEORY

The metabolic theory, also known as the rate-of-living theory, was developed by Dr. Raymond Pearl, who observed that fruit flies kept in an agitated state died much sooner than less active fruit flies. He theorized that living organisms are endowed with a certain amount of energy and that when that energy is used up, they die. Support for this theory was developed when researchers fed baby rats a nutritionally balanced diet very low in calories. The life spans of the baby rats increased by 40 percent. The theory holds that calorie deprivation causes the metabolisms of these animals to slow down, thus lengthening their life spans.

Several studies using lab animals seem to support the metabolic theory, but no studies show that calorie restriction prolongs human lives. We believe that the metabolic or rate-of-living theory has little to offer in the way of hope in prolonging people's lives. Humans aren't baby rats. Humans have free will. When we get hungry, or when we feel deprived, we eat. Often we eat too much. That's why Chapters 7, 8, and 9 discuss eating nutrient-rich, filling, antioxidant foods and provide recipes that will allow you to lose excess weight without feeling hungry.

THE GENETIC THEORY

The genetic theory says that our cells and organs are somehow programmed to self-destruct after a certain amount of time.[5] This theory states that our cells contain programmed "genetic clocks" for aging and that these genetic timepieces establish an absolute limit on how many times our cells can repair and reproduce themselves. Support for that theory appeared in the early 1960s when Dr. Leonard Hayflick, a researcher then at the University of California at San Francisco, was studying the development of fibroblasts (connective tissue cells) in a lab dish. He discovered that human cells divided only about fifty times before they wore out and died. Furthermore, Dr. Hayflick discovered that cells from older people divided fewer times and that cells from embryos divided the most. His studies provided strong support for the genetic theory of aging.[6]

Many scientists believe that the "genetic clock" may be regulated by a master hormone that influences the rate at which we age. That master hormone, melatonin, is produced by the pineal gland. As people age, levels of melatonin in their bloodstreams drop from a high of 350 units per 100 ml at two years old to levels below 30 units per 100 ml by age ninety. This dramatic drop has important ramifications. Some researchers believe that a deficiency of melatonin may be a critical starting point for a wide range of degenerative diseases.

The genetic theory has been challenged by many scientists, including Dr. Lester Packer, a professor of physiology at the University of California at Berkeley. Dr. Packer has been studying the relationships between free radicals and the aging process for about twenty-five years. A few years ago he repeated the Hayflick experiment.

However, this time Dr. Packer and his colleague, James R. Smith, used human lung cells and added vitamin E to the lab dish experiment. They then compared the vitamin E-supplemented cells to a control group of lung cells that had been treated exactly the same as those in Dr. Hayflick's original experiment. The results were eye-opening. Cells in the control culture reproduced the expected fifty times and then died. Cells in the vitamin E culture doubled more than two hundred times. *The Hayflick limit had been exceeded!* Dr. Packer concluded that the antioxidant vitamin E helped the cells remain healthy and live long beyond the fifty-replication limit.[7] More studies are needed, but this could mean that the human genetic program for aging can be rewritten and that antioxidants, especially vitamin E, provide the essential code for that revision! Dr. Packer's study provides evidence that even *if* we are genetically programmed for aging, vitamin E can still enhance good health and prolong life, perhaps by rewriting our genetic programming.

THE WEAR-AND-TEAR, FREE RADICAL THEORY

The most popular current theory of aging is the wear-and-tear theory, which holds that aging is caused by free radical reactions.[8] "There is a substantial amount of experimental evidence indicating a role for oxygen free radicals in the aging process and the development of several chronic diseases among the elderly,"[9] agrees Dr. Jeffrey Blumberg, chief of the Antioxidants Research Laboratory Tufts University and associate director of the U.S. Department of Agriculture's USDA Human Nutrition Research Center at Tufts University, Boston.

The wear-and-tear theory argues that aging results from an accumulation of oxidative stress caused by free radical damage to cells, tissues, and "all human systems."[10] Indeed, free radicals appear to be virtual wrecking balls within human bodies. In atherosclerosis, for instance, free radicals appear to injure low-density lipoproteins. In cancer, free radicals activate or "turn on" certain types of carcinogens. We will further detail the role of free radicals in coronary diseases and cancer in Chapters 3 and 4.

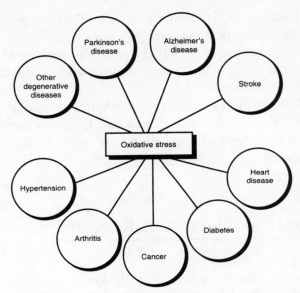

FIGURE 2.1   *Disease states and mechanism of cell death thought to be associated with oxidative stress*

Medical evidence also has shown that free radical damage is involved in several other diseases, including arthritis.[11] Arthritis causes inflammation. During inflammation, prostaglandins important to the body's defenses against injury are produced. However, the manufacture of these prostaglandins is a two-edged sword because free radicals, which cause some of the inflammatory damage of arthritis, are also formed.

Free radical damage to the pancreas is also believed to set the stage for diabetes (an impaired ability to metabolize sugar). One of the reasons diabetes occurs is that free radicals attack and damage the beta cells responsible for producing insulin. Free radicals are involved not only in the development of diabetes but also in triggering other illnesses associated with impaired sugar metabolism, such as blindness.

Free radicals are also able to cross the brain-blood barrier to harm neurons in the brain, thus hastening the aging of the brain and possibly contributing to such degenerative afflictions as Alzheimer's and

Parkinson's diseases. According to a current theory, people develop Parkinson's disease because some of the enzymes in the mitochondria generate too many free radicals, and those destroyers "kill nerve cells in the part of the brain that controls smooth and coordinated movement of muscles."[12]

Indeed, free radical reactions are so ubiquitous that, as Dr. Packer picturesquely says, "Through free radical reactions in our body, it's as though we're being irradiated at low levels all the time. They grind us down."[13]

ANTIOXIDANTS TO THE RESCUE

Many studies have linked the low intake of antioxidants to high rates of those diseases.[14] For example, clinical investigations have shown that patients suffering from Alzheimer's disease have low blood levels of antioxidants.[15] Our antiaging, antioxidant health program can help you attain a prolonged, healthy, functional life and reduce your risk for the most commonly feared chronic degenerative diseases of aging, including the senile dementia of Alzheimer's[16] and other disorders such as Parkinson's.[17]

Many other experts, including University of Kentucky colleagues Charles D. Smith, a neurologist, and John M. Carney, a pharmacologist, both at the university's Sanders-Brown Center on Aging, agree that "the cause of aging is free radical reactions on the cellular level" and that Alzheimer's disease has "features consistent with the free radical oxidation hypothesis."[18] Dr. J. Stephen Richardson, a Canadian pharmacologist, stated that "the nerve cell degeneration of Alzheimer's disease is exactly what we would expect from the action of free radicals."[19]

Because antioxidants sponge up corrosive free radicals, one way to combat the diseases of aging is to increase our intake of these life-prolonging substances. Various studies have conclusively shown that individuals who eat diets rich in antioxidants have lower mortality rates from cancer and cardiovascular problems. For instance, a

Harvard study of 87,245 female nurses published in the prestigious *New England Journal of Medicine* reported that women ages thirty-four to fifty-nine, who took vitamin E supplements for at least two years lowered their risk of heart attack almost by half.[20] Another Harvard study reported in the same issue showed a 37 percent risk reduction for men who took vitamin E.[21] In Chapters 3 and 4 we detail the role antioxidants have in protecting us from those two dread diseases.

STRENGTHEN YOUR IMMUNE SYSTEM

Antioxidants not only protect us against coronary disease and cancer, they also protect us from an assortment of other degenerative and infectious diseases. Studies by Canadian researcher Dr. Ranjit K. Chandra show how important it is to take antioxidants. He conducted what others have called a "breakthrough study" on the effects of vitamin and trace-element supplementation on the immune responses and infection rates of a group of elderly people. Roughly one-third of the subjects in his study were found to have nutrition deficiencies. This wasn't surprising. Many research studies have shown that the elderly are deficient in the antioxidant vitamins C and E, yet because their immune systems are weakening, their requirements for these vitamins are higher than the currently recommended dietary allowances. The elderly aren't the only ones at risk. Most middle-aged and younger individuals don't get enough antioxidants from their daily diets. Large-scale food consumption surveys of Americans' eating habits reveal that "very few individuals in the United States even approach the recommended levels of intake."[22]

To test the effects of increased antioxidant consumption, Dr. Chandra provided half of the study participants supplements of vitamins A, thiamine, riboflavin, niacin, B_6, folic acid, B_{12}, C, and D and the minerals iron, zinc, copper, selenium, iodine, calcium, and magnesium. Their recommended daily dose of vitamin E and beta-carotene was quadrupled. The other half of the participants in Dr. Chandra's study did *not* receive supplemental vitamins and minerals. Instead they received placebos, capsules that looked like they contained those nutrients. After one year, Dr. Chandra discovered that those who received the vitamin/mineral supplements "had significant improvement" in immune system strength. Tests proved that the individuals who took capsules containing vitamins and minerals "were less likely than those in the placebo group to have illness due to infections."[23]

Dr. Chandra's study was a breakthrough, explains Dr. Jeffrey Blumberg, a top nutrition expert at Tufts University, because it produced an impressive advance in knowledge. "Earlier studies of dietary supplementation demonstrated improvements in certain measures of immune function, but this is the first study to demonstrate improvement in a clinical sense. Patients receiving the supplements came down with fewer infectious diseases."[24]

Dr. Chandra believes that his study's findings are "of considerable clinical and public-health importance"[25] because they suggest that nutritionally deficient individuals can strengthen their immune systems and protect against infection by getting enough vitamins and minerals through supplementation.

WHAT OTHER EXPERTS SAY ABOUT ANTIOXIDANT PROTECTION

"Appropriate dietary intervention can improve immune responsiveness and reduce the burden of illness," states longtime free radical researcher Dr. Simin Nikbin Meydani and colleagues at the USDA's Human Nutrition Research Center on Aging at Tufts University, Medford, Massachusetts.[26]

"Improved immunity will lead to fewer infections," agrees Dr. John Bogden, professor of preventive medicine and community health at New Jersey Medical School. Dr. Bogden led a one-year study of twenty-nine people, all over age sixty, who took a daily multivitamin containing antioxidants. Skin tests after the study showed they had significantly healthier immune systems than did 27 others who took a placebo.[27]

Anthony T. Diplock, a biochemist at the University of London's Guy's Hospital, writes, "Evidence exists in the medical literature which, taken together, begins to make an overwhelming case for the existence of a relationship between high blood levels of antioxidant nutrients and a lowered incidence of disease."[28]

No less an authority than Dr. Kenneth H. Cooper, author of two national best-sellers—*Aerobics* and *Controlling Cholesterol*—and founder of the world-famous Cooper Aerobic Center, now believes in the protective effects of antioxidants. In his 1994 book *The Antioxidant Revolution*, Dr. Cooper states, "The latest research shows that to build strong protection against free radicals, you need to take far larger amounts of antioxidants than the official RDAs provide."[29]

TO SUM UP

• Strong evidence shows that the regular use of antioxidants can result in a longer, healthier life.

• No matter which theory of aging is correct—and aging is such a complicated process that many mechanisms are probably at work—increasing your antioxidant intake can help prevent premature aging and provide protection against degenerative diseases.

• It's best to eat a diet rich in antioxidants—at least five servings of fruits and leafy green vegetables daily. Since our busy schedules often interfere with this goal, the antioxidant supplements recommended later in this book can serve as a type of "life insurance" to help you survive longer and healthier.

HAZEL TURNS NINETY

To close this chapter, let's look at Hazel, who at age ninety, is still going strong. She celebrated her ninetieth birthday in November 1995. Her two daughters, five grandchildren, and eleven great-grandchildren all gathered to help her celebrate. Hazel retired at age sixty-five to travel with her first husband but, after his death, served as a church secretary for five years, finally retiring at age seventy-five. At the same time, she maintained her own eleven-room home with opulent gardens. She did most of the gardening herself! Almost annually her home was in the *Showcase of Homes* or the *Parade of Gardens*. Just before her last birthday, Hazel announced to her Sunday school class that she was retiring as their teacher, since the print of the teaching materials was now too small for her to read easily. The wonder is that she had taught that class as long as she had, some fifty years! It had become known as "Hazel's class."

Everyone realizes that Hazel is a remarkable woman. She has an adventuresome spirit that surprises her teenage great-grandchildren. Fewer than ten years ago she could still outhike her children and grandchildren. She continues to be interested in learning new things. In the past decade she has completed and published three books: a family history, an anecdotal history of her early years, and a book of poetry. She remains actively interested in her extended family. She remains the one whom family members call on for advice.

About ten years ago Hazel came to see Dr. Anderson because of newly discovered diabetes. (As we age, we do become more prone to degenerative diseases.) She also had high triglyceride levels. Up to then, Hazel had followed the typical high-fat, low-fiber American diet. When she learned of our program, she enthusiastically began to follow its dietary principles and added regular walks to her active lifestyle. Her triglyceride levels came down to more normal levels.

For about seven years, she was able to successfully manage her diabetic condition with diet, antidiabetes pills, and low-intensity exercise, mostly walking. Although she eventually had to go on insulin, we were all surprised that she had been able to delay doing so as long as she had.

Three years ago Dr. Anderson was just starting to put patients on the antioxidant regimen. Hazel was one of the first to try it. She soon reported that the antioxidant-rich foods and supplements gave her an energy boost. It must still be working. She still continues to manage her own home and give advice about many aspects of life to her children, grandchildren, and great-grandchildren. When they have a puzzling problem, "Nana" is the first person they call on.

I feel that the antioxidant program, combined with Hazel's upbeat attitude, active lifestyle, commitment to learning, willingness to try new ways, and her family's emotional support, have helped her survive to enjoy her later years. I fully expect Hazel to continue on the antioxidant, antiaging program and become one of the million or so individuals who achieve the century mark in age.

3

GAIN PROTECTION AGAINST HEART DISEASE AND STROKE

ROBERT FIGHTS HEART DISEASE, LOWERS BLOOD CHOLESTEROL AND SUGAR LEVELS

Robert is an energetic salesman and biker who looks younger than his sixty-five years. He came to my office in 1990 because of diabetes and high blood cholesterol levels. He owned a bike shop until two years previously, when he was shocked by an unexpected heart attack. At that time Robert was twenty pounds overweight, and his diabetes and high blood cholesterol conditions had just been discovered. He became depressed, sold his bicycle shop, and settled into a couch-potato existence. After watching me being interviewed by a TV reporter, Robert asked for my help in controlling his medical conditions.

Robert's treatment program included the antioxidant food plan and an antioxidant "cocktail" supplement of beta-carotene, vitamin C, and vitamin E. He quickly lost fifteen pounds, and his blood glucose and blood cholesterol levels dropped dramatically. He resumed biking and achieved a level of fitness and vigor he had not enjoyed for fifteen years. Robert returned to his former bike shop, to the delight of the new owner, and became a supersalesman. Today he is at his ideal weight, is robust, cycles six to eight miles per day, and has no evidence of coronary heart disease. Tests of the fat particles (lipids) in his bloodstream show that he has less risk for a heart attack and stroke than most men twenty years younger.

TABLE 3.1 ROBERT'S SCORECARD

MEASUREMENT	INITIAL VALUE	THREE-MONTH VALUE	THREE-YEAR VALUE	GOALS
Cholesterol	250*	216	191	≤200
LDL cholesterol	184*	161	99	≤100
HDL cholesterol	42*	42	46	≥ 45
Triglycerides	158*	67	136	≤150
Glucose	186*	156	122	≤140

* All values are for mg/100 ml.

THE KEY TO AVOIDING HEART DISEASE

Like Robert, almost 5 million Americans have heart attacks each year. Almost 1 million die from cardiovascular disease, including heart attacks, strokes, and other circulation problems. Most of us have relatives or friends with diagnosed or undiagnosed heart disease. This silent killer strikes at the prime of life, when you and your loved ones should be spending more time traveling, improving golf scores, and enjoying grandchildren. Since three-quarters of all heart attacks are preventable, these are distressing death statistics. Like Robert, you probably want to reduce your risk for heart attack and help friends and family members do the same. This book gives you the tools to achieve both goals. Put into practice the advice contained here, and share it with others. You can change the odds, tilting them in your favor.

New research has shown that avoiding a heart attack isn't just a matter of avoiding high cholesterol and saturated fat foods such as eggs, butter, and prime ribs. You can also reduce the risk of heart disease by eating antioxidant-rich vegetables and fruits and by taking antioxidant supplements. If you couple this with regular exercise and refrain from smoking, you will enjoy a longer, healthier life. This antioxidant program will nip hardening of the arteries in the bud. It will reverse the process of arteriosclerosis (artery hardening) and even demolish blockages that are already present.

WHAT THIS CHAPTER DOES

This chapter explains new insights about how free radicals contribute to the process that leads to heart attacks and strokes. We will tell you about some of the research that led to these insights and then tell you how to get your own antioxidant program into high gear.

HOW HEART ATTACKS REALLY OCCUR

The accumulation of cholesterol in blood vessel walls plays a critical role in the process that leads to heart attacks and strokes. Free radical oxidation of fat particles in the blood contributes to the process of cholesterol accumulation. This process, known as hardening of the arteries (arteriosclerosis), leads to heart attacks and strokes. The process is the same for both conditions. However, if it occurs in a coronary artery, it can lead to a heart attack. If it occurs in a cerebral artery, an artery leading to the brain, the result can be a stroke.

New research indicates that heart attacks and strokes occur because blood vessels rupture and leak a fatty gruel, which leads to formation of a blood clot that completely blocks or closes off the blood vessel. The blood vessels rupture because of a buildup of internal pressure that occurs after a chain of circumstances with free radicals at its start. Here's what happens.

We ingest cholesterol and fat in our daily diet, but our body also manufactures fat and cholesterol. We've heard so many negatives about these substances that many people don't realize they also serve positive purposes. Fat stores energy, acts as insulation to protect the body against the stress of cold environments, and also serves as a shock absorber for our internal organs. Cholesterol is a precursor or building block for the creation of bile acids needed for digestion and for the generation of hormones that regulate metabolism, growth, and reproduction.

Fat and cholesterol in the bloodstream are called lipids. Together with protein they are called lipoproteins. There are several types of lipoproteins, depending on how tightly packed they are. There are low-density lipoproteins (LDLs), high-density lipoproteins (HDLs), and very-low-density lipoproteins (VLDLs). To make it easier to write about these substances, the medical literature usually refers to lipoproteins by those abbreviations without the small "s," as if they were singular rather than plural. In addition, both LDL and HDL have nicknames. LDL has been nicknamed "bad guy" cholesterol because, when LDL reaches a certain threshold level in the bloodstream, it squeezes between the outer cell walls (endothelial linings) of a blood vessel (either coronary or cerebral) and takes up residence there (see Figure 3.1). During this journey, the LDL "bad guys" are attacked by free radicals and oxidized—that is, they become "rusty." This "rust" is then engulfed by macrophages, which are protector cells in the blood vessel walls. Remember the story from ancient history about how the Greeks conquered the city of Troy by constructing a giant, hollow figure of a horse in which a troop of Greek soldiers hid? The Trojans rolled the "horse" within the protecting walls of their city, and later that night the Greek soldiers escaped from their concealment and opened the city gates. Similarly, when the macrophage protector cells are stuffed full of rusty LDL, they no longer act to defend the cell wall. In fact, they are stuck within it. Ironically, they then become Trojan horse menaces called foam cells.

Foam cells are packed with fat and get their name from the foamy sheen of the many fat droplets they carry. Relatively speaking, these foam cells become enormous, at least in comparison to the microscopic world within an artery that they inhabit. Because of their large size they can no longer move. Like couch potatoes, they just lie within the blood vessel wall, holding as much fat as they can.

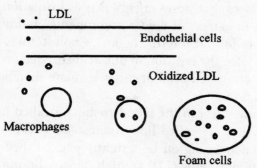

FIGURE 3.1   *This figure illustrates the process by which LDL enter the blood vessel wall, are oxidized to rusty LDL and then taken up by macrophages which are converted to foam cells, the earliest lesions of arteriosclerosis.*

When the blood vessel becomes crowded with foam cells it develops a yellow, streaky appearance. This is the earliest stage of arteriosclerosis. As this process continues, more foam cells and fat accumulate, forming a protrusion or bump extending out from the blood vessel wall. This is termed an atheroma. Because antioxidants do not penetrate atheromas very well, free radicals have a field day. They oxidize all the LDL in reach. The rusty LDL is rapidly sucked up by other foam cells, which causes the creation of new atheromas and the growth of others. Little atheromas coalesce to become big atheromas. This process damages blood vessels because, as an atheroma grows larger, it puts strain on and weakens the wall of the blood vessel where it is located. Like a large pimple, it may rupture when traumatized by an increase in blood pressure or when the blood vessel dilates to accommodate increased blood flow.[1] Fibrotic scar tissue forms at the site of this repeated injury. Medical scientists have characterized this point in the process of arteriosclerosis as midstage.

Let's recap, since it is a complicated process. As a result of foam cell buildup, the blood vessel becomes narrower. Large, mushy atheromas develop, which impede or partially block blood flow. Most heart attacks occur because of the rupture of one of the large, mushy atheromas. Recent studies have shown that the site of rup-

Clot formation

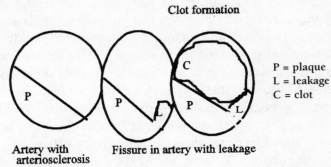

P = plaque
L = leakage
C = clot

**Artery with
arteriosclerosis**   **Fissure in artery with leakage**

FIGURE 3.2   *This drawing illustrates the process of blood clot formation in a blood vessel with existing arteriosclerosis.*

ture always has an enormous accumulation of foam cells pressing on it, leading to weakness in the blood vessel wall. Realize that the rupture begins as the result of free radical bombardment of LDL at the blood vessel wall. The free radicals are engulfed by protector cells which, when engorged, turn into "Trojan horse" atheromas, dangerous tubs of lard within the artery wall. By their expanding presence, atheromas put pressure on the blood vessel walls. They also weaken those walls by protruding into the channel through which blood flows. The channel narrows, causing the rushing blood to fill every space, putting further pressure on the weakened artery wall. Like the Greek soldiers hidden in the Trojan horse who opened the city gates, the atheromas open holes in the cell wall.

In the human body, however, the process does not have to in-

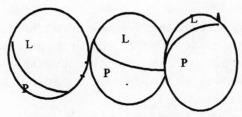

P= plaque; L= lumen of blood vessel

FIGURE 3.3   *Progressive narrowing of blood vessel due to arteriosclerosis.*

evitably lead to rupture. If the Trojans had had reinforcements, their city might not have fallen. We can provide our body with reinforcements of vitamin E and vitamin C. Vitamin E molecules join the defensive combat as free radical scavengers, attacking and destroying free radical demons without becoming devils themselves—that is, without becoming foam cells. Vitamin E can do this because it is constantly being "refreshed"—that is, repaired—by vitamin C. Research indicates that vitamin C, at least in this process, doesn't appear to directly engage the free radical/rusty LDL enemy directly. Instead, it supports its loyal buddy, vitamin E, as a sort of paramedic. Vitamin E attacks rusty LDL by crumbling it up, letting it wash away in the bloodstream. This prevents the buildup of foam cells, stops the formation of atheromas, and breaks the chain of events that causes coronary heart attack or, in a cerebral artery, stroke.

Understanding this process can lead to better prevention. Since fat-laden foam cells have their start when LDL cholesterol is oxidized, it makes sense to take steps to reduce LDL levels. That's where a low-fat diet, high in antioxidants, comes in. The antioxidants in food are digested and sent into the bloodstream to take their place in the ongoing battle. High antioxidant intake means decreased oxidative damage to LDL and a lowered risk for heart disease and stroke.

HOW ANTIOXIDANTS PREVENT LDL OXIDATION

Let's now review the research evidence that allowed us to figure out the disease process described above. For instance, what evidence do we have to support our conclusion that antioxidants such as vitamin E slow the process of hardening of the arteries by blocking LDL oxidation?

ANTIOXIDANT STUDIES IN ANIMALS

Animal studies show that supplementing the diet with antioxidants significantly decreases the development of arteriosclerosis in those animals fed high-fat and high-cholesterol diets. These animals develop severe arteriosclerosis when they are fed unhealthy diets. Several different antioxidants, including vitamin E, decrease the development of atherosclerosis. These studies indicate that the rate of narrowing of blood vessels is reduced by 50 percent to 80 percent. Because different types of antioxidants have been used, the effect appears to be directly related to the free radical scavenging properties of those antioxidants.[2]

ANTIOXIDANT STUDIES IN HUMANS

Our research group at the VA Medical Center in Lexington, Kentucky, recently published results of a study that shows that daily use of antioxidant supplements significantly decreases oxidation of LDL in the blood of diabetic men. As you may know, diabetics have roughly twice the risk of heart attacks than nondiabetics. Every day for twelve weeks, the diabetic men took the following antioxidant supplements: beta-carotene, 24,000 units (14.4 mg); vitamin C, 1,000 mg; and vitamin E, 800 units (800 mg). After twelve weeks, samples of their blood were taken and the rate of oxidation of the LDL of their blood was measured. Before treatment, the time required for oxidation of LDL from the men was forty-two minutes. After twelve weeks of antioxidant supplementation, the oxidation time increased significantly, to ninety minutes, more than a twofold increase. In other words, the men had twice as much protection from free radicals after taking the antioxidant supplements as they had before the study.

STUDIES BY OTHER EXPERTS

You may be wondering, "What are the benefits of this demonstration?" Studies from other laboratories document that the LDL oxidation time (technically, the lag phase for oxidation) is inversely related to presence of heart disease. An inverse relationship is like a playground teeter-totter. When one end goes up, the other goes down. Thus those individuals whose LDL is rapidly oxidized in the test tube have much more extensive heart disease than those whose LDL is resistant to oxidation.[3] You and I would rather have very slowly oxidized LDL to reduce our risk of heart disease.

TABLE 3.2   STUDIES ASSOCIATING HIGH INTAKE OF ANTIOXIDANT VITAMINS WITH REDUCED RISK OF CORONARY HEART DISEASE (CHD)

Study	Antioxidant Vitamin	Reduction in Risk
Gey[4]	Vitamin E blood level (high vs. low)	CHD deaths were 83% lower
Riemersma[5]	Vitamin E blood level (high vs. low)	Angina was 63% lower
Stampfer[7]	Vitamin E intake (high vs. low)	CHD deaths were 46% lower
Rimm[6]	Vitamin E intake (high vs. low)	CHD deaths were 37% lower
Kardinaal[8]	Beta-carotene level in fatty tissue (high vs. low)	Heart attacks were 58% lower among smokers
Rimm[6]	Beta-carotene intake (high vs. low)	CHD deaths were 40% lower among former smokers
Gaziano[9]	Beta-carotene supplements (high vs. low)	Heart attacks were 51% lower
Gaziano[10]	Beta-carotene intake (high vs. low)	CHD deaths were 68% lower
Morris[11]	Carotenoid blood level (high vs. low)	Heart attacks were 36% lower
Street[12]	Carotenoid blood level (high vs. low)	Heart attacks were 56% lower
Enstrom[13]	Vitamin C intake (high vs. low)	CHD deaths were lower

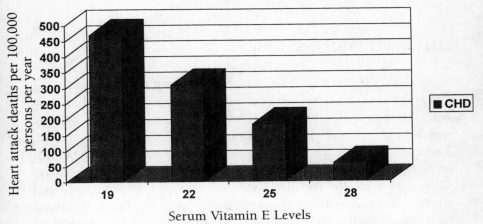

FIGURE 3.4   *Serum vitamin E and risk for heart attack.*

Table 3.2 summarizes some of the studies examining the relationship between antioxidant vitamin intake and rates of CHD and heart attacks. As illustrated in Figure 3.4, the pioneering studies of Dr. K. F. Gey[4] documented that heart attacks are more common in Finland than in Spain. Why? In an attempt to answer the question, he conducted what became a landmark study. He discovered that blood levels of vitamin E are inversely related to rates of heart attack across sixteen different European countries. Remember, an inverse relationship is like a playground teeter-totter. When one end goes up, the other goes down. In countries such as Spain, where blood levels of vitamin E are high, rates of heart attack are low. In contrast, in countries such as Finland, where blood levels of vitamin E levels are low, heart attack rates are high. More than a dozen studies indicate that high intakes of antioxidant vitamins are associated with lower rates of heart attack. In the Spain versus Finland population study, the Spanish population, which had the highest vitamin E blood levels, had an 83 percent *lower* rate of heart attack than the Finnish population, with the lowest vitamin E blood levels.

OTHER VITAMIN E STUDIES

Similarly, another study[5] found that Scottish men with the highest vitamin E blood levels had a 63 percent lower rate of angina than men with the lowest vitamin E blood levels. In separate studies of large numbers of men and of women, Drs. E. B. Rimm[6] and M. J. Stampfer[7] found that persons who took vitamin E supplements had 37 percent to 46 percent fewer heart attacks than persons with the lowest level of vitamin E intake. Dr. Rimm studied vitamin E consumption and the risk of coronary heart disease in a large sample, of forty thousand men. Dr. Stampfer studied vitamin E consumption and the risk of coronary disease in a sample of more than eighty thousand women who took at least and often more than 100 IU per day of vitamin E for more than two years. It was this group that showed the 46 percent lower risk of heart disease. These three studies strongly suggest that regular intake of vitamin E supplements reduces risk for heart attack.

BETA-CAROTENE

Beta-carotene also appears to reduce heart attack risk. Dr. A. F. M. Kardinaal[8] and colleagues measured beta-carotene content in fatty tissue of smokers to estimate the level of that substance prior to intake of beta-carotene. Those with the highest fatty tissue levels of beta-carotene had a 58 percent lower rate of heart attack than smokers with fatty tissue with the lowest beta-carotene levels. In a study of a large number of men, Dr. Rimm[6] found that the highest level of beta-carotene intake was associated with a 40 percent lower rate of heart attack among former smokers than among smokers with low levels of beta-carotene.

Researchers[9, 10] have shown that a group of subjects with the highest level of beta-carotene intake had a 51 percent to 68 percent lower rate of heart attack or death from heart attack than a group of similar subjects with low levels of beta-carotene. Two other studies[11, 12] examined the total amount of carotenoids in the blood.[11] Both found that people with the highest levels of blood carotenoids had 36 percent to 56 percent lower rates of heart attack than people with the lowest levels of blood carotenoids. The number of studies with consistently similar results suggests that a high intake of beta-carotene from carrots, sweet potatoes, or vegetable juice—or use of beta-carotene supplements—reduces the risk of heart attack. To learn more about beta-carotene, see the section "The Great Vitamin Scares of 1994 and 1996" starting on page 64.

VITAMIN C

The effects of vitamin C intake on risk of heart attack are less persuasive. Vitamin C, being water-soluble, is not transported by LDL. Thus it is not carried into the blood vessel wall to protect the LDL there from vicious attack by free radicals. Nevertheless, as previously pointed out, research does show that vitamin C works like a blocker in a football game, protecting the quarterback, vitamin E, from damage. Vitamin C even acts as a paramedic and restores vitamin E to full strength after it is damaged by free radicals. In that way, generous intakes of vitamin C can be said to reduce risk for heart attack. If this is true, researchers should be able to show an association between vitamin C intake and lower levels of heart disease. Indeed, a large epidemiological study of vitamin C intake in a U.S. population sample by Dr. J. E. Enstrom[13] suggests that high levels of vitamin C intake are associated with lower rates of death from coronary heart disease.

OTHER ANTIOXIDANTS

Like vitamins C and E and beta-carotene, there are many other important antioxidants in the diet. Flavonoids are antioxidant substances found in many vegetables, fruits, and beverages such as tea and red wine. These compounds affect the color and flavor of these foods. Hertog[14] has carefully measured the various flavonoids in the Dutch diet. He reports that the diets of elderly Dutch men with high flavonoid intake, largely provided by tea, onions, and apples, was associated with a 68 percent lower rate of death from heart attack than for men with a low intake of flavonoids. These studies are consistent with other reports that intake of red wine or green tea, both rich in flavonoids, is associated with a lower rate of heart attack.[15]

OTHER IMPORTANT VITAMINS (THE FABB STORY)

Recent research indicates that a high blood level of homocysteine, an important amino acid or building block of protein, may contribute to heart attack or stroke in certain people.[16] At high blood levels homocysteine is toxic to the endothelial lining of the flat cells on the outer layer of blood vessels. It may also increase blood clotting, thereby setting the stage for heart attack or stroke.

Elevated blood levels of homocysteine have been linked to intake of three water-soluble vitamins: folic acid, vitamin B_6, and vitamin B_{12} (FABB). The intake of higher amounts of these three vitamins decreases homocysteine in blood to the normal range.[17] Since people at high risk for heart attack or stroke have higher blood levels of homocysteine than persons at low risk, these data seem to indicate a benefit for taking that trio of B vitamins. Furthermore, other studies indicate that people who develop circulation problems before age fifty are very likely to have high blood levels of homocysteine and develop premature blood vessel disease. *Consequently, persons with parents or siblings with premature blood vessel disease should daily take 1 mg of folic acid, 25 mg of vitamin B_6, and 10 mg of vitamin B_{12} orally.* Because homocysteine levels are also increased in many persons with hardening of the arteries, we recommend that all individuals already diagnosed with heart disease, cerebral vascular disease, or other circulation problems take these supplements daily.

THE "GOOD GUY" VERSUS THE "BAD GUY" CHOLESTEROL REVISITED

As we have seen, LDL, the "bad guy" low-density lipoprotein, is the most important risk factor for arteriosclerosis. Similarly, oxidation of LDL by free radicals is strongly related to hardening of the arteries. Other factors also contribute. High-density lipoproteins (HDL), the "good guys," have a very important protective function. HDL prevents oxidation of LDL and even repairs free radical-damaged LDL. HDL also acts like an avenging vampire, extracting cholesterol from foam cells in an attempt to restore these damaged cells to health. While high blood LDL levels are the worst risk factor for arteriosclerosis, high blood HDL levels are the best. Low-fat, high-fiber diets lower your LDL, while healthy habits such as exercise and smoking avoidance raise your HDL.

Most laboratory tests of human blood are done after a twelve-hour fast. Lab tests are usually done to measure the amount of LDL, HDL, and VLDL. This third lipoprotein carries most of the triglycerides in the blood. Triglycerides are composed of three ("tri-") fatty acids linked to a small glycerol (glyceride) molecule. Triglycerides are produced in the liver and are also made in the intestines after a meal. After a meal, the intestines package dietary fatty acids and cholesterol into chylomicrons (fatty particles). As these chylomicrons enter the bloodstream, they raise the triglyceride content for six to ten hours. Chylomicrons are the fourth major fat particle in the blood. As indicated, HDL protect against arteriosclerosis. However, LDL, VLDL, and breakdown products of chylomicrons *contribute to arteriosclerosis.*

Although our bodies manufacture triglycerides, most of those fat molecules get into our bloodstream from the fat in the meat, cheese, and dressings we eat. That's why we should minimize our fat intake. It reduces our risk for developing arteriosclerosis.

TABLE 3.3   DESIRABLE SERUM LIPID LEVELS; VALUES ARE IN MG/100 ML

MEASURE	GENERAL PREVENTIVE*	TAILORED PROTECTION	DISEASE REVERSAL
Cholesterol	<240	<200	<170
LDL cholesterol	<160	<130	<100
HDL cholesterol	> 35	> 45 for men	> 45 for men
		> 55 for women	> 55 for women
Triglycerides	<250	<150	<100

* General preventive values are recommendations for persons without risk factors for coronary heart disease. Tailored protection recommendations are for persons with risk factors for coronary heart disease. Disease reversal recommendations are for persons with established coronary heart disease.

Table 3.3 outlines desirable blood fat levels. All adults should have blood serum levels in the general preventive range indicated in that table. Persons with risk factors as outlined in Table 3.4 should have serum lipids in the tailored protection range. If someone has a diagnosis of coronary heart disease, serum lipids should be in the disease reversal range. As a general rule, children should have serum cholesterol values of <170, LDL cholesterol values of fewer than 100, HDL cholesterol values of more than 50, and triglycerides of fewer than 150 mg/100 ml.

TABLE 3.4   NONLIPID RISK FACTORS FOR CORONARY HEART DISEASE

Risk Factor	Desirable Value	Relative Risk*
High systolic blood pressure	<120 mm Hg	To 3.3 (men)
		To 4.4 (women)
Cigarette smoking	No	To 4.0
Diabetes	No	To 2.6 (men)
		To 4.6 (women)
Obesity	Nonobese	To 2.2
Inactivity	Active	To 3.2
High serum fibrinogen level	<180 mg/dl	To 4.0 (men)
		To 10.7 (women)
High serum uric acid level	<4.0 mg/dl	To 2.0
High serum homocysteine level	Variable	Unknown
Low vitamin E intake	400 IU daily	To 1.7
Poor stress management	Not delineated	Unknown

*Relative risk represents highest risk for highly abnormal values. For example, with the highest blood pressure category, the risk for heart attack is 3.3 times (330 percent) higher than for the lowest blood pressure category. Values are given for men or women if there are known differences for risks for the sexes. Modified from Anderson.[18]

NONLIPID RISK FACTORS

Although abnormalities of LDL and its oxidation are important contributors to the arteriosclerosis process, other risk factors also contribute to coronary heart disease. Table 3.4 summarizes these nonlipid risk factors. The major three risk factors for coronary heart disease are high LDL cholesterol, high blood pressure, and cigarette smoking. These risk factors can increase for one's chances of heart attack by up to four times. Other risk factors are as follows:

- Diabetes is a much greater risk factor for women than for men. The reasons for this difference are unknown.
- Obesity and inactivity are also obvious and significant risk factors.
- High fibrinogen levels in the blood enhance clotting and thus promote formation of blood clots in blood vessels. Daily intake of aspirin reduces the effects of high fibrinogen levels.
- High serum uric acid levels also increase the risk of heart attack.
- As discussed above, low intake of vitamin E and high-serum homocysteine levels are newly identified risk factors.
- Finally, poor management of stress sets the stage for heart attack.

HOW THE ANTIOXIDANT, ANTIAGING PROGRAM COMBATS HEART DISEASE

Your antioxidant program is a comprehensive approach to reducing your risk for developing heart disease, stroke, or other blood vessel diseases. If you already have evidence of some arteriosclerosis, this program will stop the process dead and begin reversing it. Your antioxidant food plan in Chapter 8 outlines quick and easy ways to enjoy healthy eating. In addition to its high antioxidant content, this food plan is rich in complex carbohydrates and dietary fibers and low in saturated fats and cholesterol. It emphasizes monounsaturated fats such as canola oil or olive oil. The health benefits of soy protein are outlined in Chapter 7, and the importance of using supplemental antioxidant vitamins is also explained in Chapter 8. You will find that Table 8.1 in Chapter 8 gives you a bird's-eye view of the entire program.

An ideal preventive program for arteriosclerosis should do the following:

- lower LDL;
- raise HDL;
- lower triglycerides;
- lower blood pressure;
- lower blood glucose;
- decrease blood clotting;
- assist in weight maintenance.

Our research over the past twenty years and the research cited in this chapter document that your antioxidant program will do these things. What we can't measure is the shrinking of the atheromas in the blood vessels. But recent research in animals and humans indicates that this shrinking is taking place, so we believe that if you embark on this program, you will benefit from a steady reversal of any arteriosclerosis you have.

TO SUM UP

- Hardening of the arteries (arteriosclerosis) includes atheroma formation in blood vessels and narrowing of blood vessels.
- LDL accumulation and damage by free radicals play a central role in this process.
- Animal studies show that administration of antioxidants such as vitamin E reduce the rate of progression of arteriosclerotic lesions.
- Human studies indicate that high levels of antioxidant intake, especially vitamin E, reduce risk of heart attack by about 50 percent.

This evidence strongly suggests that the use of an antioxidant-rich diet and antioxidant supplements should significantly decrease your risk of developing heart attack or stroke.

WHAT YOU CAN DO NOW

GENERAL PREVENTION

If you are in good health and do not have any of the risk factors listed in Table 3.4, you still want to reduce your risk of developing a heart attack.

- Have your serum cholesterol, LDL cholesterol, HDL cholesterol, and triglycerides measured to see whether you are in the desirable range given in Table 3.3.
- Begin the antioxidant diet and exercise program summarized in the left-hand column in Table 8.1.
- Start taking one multivitamin-mineral capsule, two antioxidant capsules, and one enteric-coated aspirin (coated to prevent stomach irritation) per day.
- Begin addressing the other health-promoting behaviors listed in Table 8.1.

TAILORED PROTECTION

If you have a strong family history of heart disease, strokes, or blood vessel disease, *or* if you have one or more risk factors listed in Table 3.4, you will want to begin the antioxidant program as soon as possible to reduce your risk of heart disease.

- Have your serum cholesterol, LDL cholesterol, HDL cholesterol, and triglycerides measured to see whether you are in the desirable range given in Table 3.3.

- Begin the antioxidant diet and exercise program summarized in the center column in Table 8.1.
- Start taking one multivitamin-mineral preparation, four antioxidant supplement capsules, two fish oil capsules, and one enteric-coated aspirin daily.
- Begin addressing the other health-promoting behaviors listed in Table 8.1.

DISEASE REVERSAL

If you have evidence of arteriosclerotic disease such as angina or a previous heart attack or stroke, or if you have had diagnostic tests indicating hardening of the arteries, you probably are already doing most of these things. The following points can serve as a checklist to ensure that you are on the full antioxidant program.

- Have your serum cholesterol, LDL cholesterol, HDL cholesterol, and triglycerides measured to see whether you are in the desirable range given in the right-hand column in Table 3.3.
- Begin the antioxidant diet and exercise program summarized in the right-hand column in Table 8.1.
- Start taking one multivitamin-mineral capsule, four antioxidant capsules, and one enteric-coated aspirin per day. You also should start the FABB supplement to lower your blood homocysteine level.
- Begin seriously addressing the other health-promoting behaviors listed in Table 8.1.

JIM'S DIARY

Because our research was indicating clear benefits of antioxidant supplements, I began taking them in 1992. For about three years I took beta-carotene, 16,000 IU or 9.6 mg; vitamin C, 1,000 mg; and vitamin E, 800 IU or 800 mg, daily. In early 1995 I changed to tablets with other supplements, including selenium. At about the same time

I started seeking out antioxidant-rich foods. As outlined in Chapter 8, I use soy protein which is rich in isoflavones; green tea, brimful of flavonoids; grapes and grape juice, which teem with polyphenols; garlic and onions, which are stuffed with sulfated antioxidants; carrots and sweet potatoes, which are packed full of beta-carotene; oranges and other fruits and vegetables abundant in vitamin C; and cruciferous vegetables, which offer a variety of health-promoting phytochemicals. I really enjoy eating this wide range of foods and sharing with other people the health benefits of this food plan. Usually I embarrass my wife, Gay, when I start "lecturing" to dinner companions about the health benefits of specific foods.

PROTECT YOURSELF AGAINST CANCER

ANTIOXIDANT SUPPLEMENTS PROTECT CHINESE FROM CANCER

Linxian County in north-central China had one of the highest rates of cancer of the esophagus in the world. Death rates from this type of cancer was a hundredfold higher in this area of China than in the United States. Because fruits and vegetables appear to reduce risk for developing various types of cancer, investigators from China and the United States developed a plan to examine the effects of nutritional supplements on rates of cancer in this rural county.[1] Since the ingredients of fruits and vegetables that protect from cancer have not been identified, researchers decided to test four combinations of nutrients: (1) vitamin A and zinc; (2) riboflavin and niacin (B vitamins); (3) vitamin C and molybdenum; and (4) beta-carotene (15 mg or 25,000 IU per day), vitamin E (30 mg or 30 IU per day), and selenium (50 mcg per day).

Participants in this research study took the supplements as tablets daily for sixty-three months. Compliance was measured by counting the pills not taken and by measuring blood levels of the nutrients under study; compliance was estimated to be 93 percent of pills taken. Almost 30,000 men and women, aged forty to sixty-nine years and considered to be relatively healthy, participated in this study. Death rates from all causes, various types of cancer, cerebrovascular disease (strokes), and other causes were tabulated.

Three of the supplements did not affect death rates from any cause. However, the supplement with beta-carotene, vitamin E, and selenium significantly decreased death rates from all causes by 9 percent over five years. Death rates from all forms of cancer were 13 percent lower and death rates from stomach cancer were 21 percent lower. Death rates from lung cancer (down 45 percent) and strokes (down 10 percent) also decreased,[1] but because of the low rates of lung cancer in this area, the large reduction in death rate was not statistically significant.[2]

This important study was one of the first to carefully examine the effects of antioxidant supplementation on the risk of developing cancer. While there are many unique features about the population in this region of north-central China, the results are exciting. They suggest that the intake of generous amounts of beta-carotene, vitamin E, and selenium may reduce risk of developing several forms of cancer.

CANCER IN THE UNITED STATES— AN "UNSUCCESS" STORY

Cancer, the second leading cause of death in the United States, continues to puzzle and confound medical doctors and researchers. Each year cancer kills more than five hundred thousand people in the United States; cancer will be the leading cause of death in the United States by the year 2000. While deaths from heart attacks have decreased 45 percent in thirty years, the incidence of cancer has increased 44 percent since 1950. Breast cancer and colon cancer rates have increased 60 percent each, prostate cancer has doubled, and lung cancer has increased 262 percent. Since cigarette smoking has decreased from 50 percent to 25 percent, these increases cannot be attributed to smoking. These grim statistics indicate that if you are a woman, you have a 1.6-fold greater chance of developing breast cancer than your grandmother did, while if you are a man, you have a twofold greater risk of developing prostate cancer than your grandfather did. In the United States, we are slowly losing ground to cancer. There is no evidence that thirty-five years of intensive research and agonizing treatment procedures have decreased the pain, suffering, and death related to cancer.[3]

Many experts recommend more emphasis on prevention and less on intensive treatment.[3] There is widespread consensus among experts that about one-third of all cancers are related to what we eat. The conservative National Academy of Sciences concluded that 35 percent of cancers are related to diet.[4] Many experts feel that virtually all types of cancer, except for rare inherited forms, are related to environmental factors such as cigarette smoking, pollutants, and nutrition. While much attention has addressed food ingredients that may cause cancer (such as fat and nitrosamines), less attention has been devoted to nutrients that may protect from cancer. Recent evidence points to antioxidants and other phytochemicals as chemoprotective agents. Since rates of cancer are not declining, many experts feel that we should take aggressive measures to prevent cancers. Consequently, "chemoprevention" had emerged as a major buzzword at the National Cancer Institute.

Chemoprevention refers to supplying certain protective substances in the diet or as supplements to prevent the development of cancer. Most of the identified chemopreventive compounds are phytochemicals or chemicals found in foods. In fact, most of the chemoprotective agents have potent antioxidant activity. Certain phytochemicals block the formation of chemical carcinogens in the stomach, protect DNA and cell membranes from damage by free radicals, and enhance immune responsiveness.[5]

PHYTOCHEMICALS PHYTE MANY DISEASES

All plants contain compounds that assist in growth, protect from insects and molds, and provide color and flavor. These phytochemicals (from phyto, or plant) offer many health benefits for humans. Vitamins C and E are phytochemicals because these antioxidants originate in plants. Many phytochemicals have antioxidant or anti-inflammatory properties that offer protection against cancer, heart disease, and other conditions. More than sixty thousand phytochemicals have been identified, and more are being discovered every year. However, the health benefits of most of them have not been delineated (Appendix A, Antioxidant and Phytochemical Advisory, gives you an overview of the major phytochemical classes and compounds). It seems likely that most of the health-promoting chemicals in broccoli, for example, have not been identified. Therefore it is important to eat a wide variety of fruits and vegetables to obtain the full health-enhancing benefits that nature provides. While we recommend supplements to obtain a protective minimum of vitamins, minerals, and antioxidants, we also strongly recommend certain vegetables and fruits, such as broccoli and cantaloupe, that are rich in health-enhancing phytochemicals. These foods, abundant in beta-carotene, also are rich in other phytochemicals that likely provide very important health benefits.

WHAT ARE CHEMOPROTECTORS, AND HOW DO THEY WORK?

As mentioned in Chapter 2, the human body contains about 63 trillion cells. Each day the average human cell is bombarded by at least 10,000 free radicals. Each "hit" can lead to mutations or changes in the cell memory (DNA), which can lead to aging, cancer, or cell death. However, most of the damage is repaired by enzyme machinery in the cell, aided by antioxidants. Antioxidants and other phytochemicals act to prevent free radical damage or "hits" and then assist in repair of DNA and cell walls or membranes.[6, 7] However, unrepaired damage over time may increase the risk of cancer and contribute to aging.[7]

Antioxidants and other phytochemicals play a vital role in protecting cells from oxidative damage and even repairing damage once it has happened. In the experimental production of cancer, these three major steps have been identified: *initiation, promotion,* and *progression.* Antioxidants and other phytochemicals can act at each of these steps to prevent, slow down, or reverse the process.

INITIATION

The initiation phase of cancer begins when DNA within the cell nucleus is damaged by a free radical, toxic chemical, irradiation, or virus. If this damage is unrepaired the cell may die, become prematurely aged, or become a precancerous cell. Antioxidants and phytochemicals can protect the cell from damage by these toxic factors by inactivating them or repairing the damage; they also may increase the enzyme machinery responsible for protecting or repairing cell components. Enhancing immune function also would reduce risk from damage from viruses. Beta-carotene and vitamin E, as lipid soluble antioxidants, protect lipid membranes from becoming oxidized. Vitamin C acts in part to regenerate vitamin E after it has been damaged by free radicals. Both vitamins C and E have a preinitiation protective function in preventing formation of nitrosamines in the stomach and thus reducing risk of stomach cancer.[8, 9]

PROMOTION

The promotion phase involves converting the initiated cell into a precancerous cell. Since there usually is a long latent or dormant period, this is a long-term process that has great potential for intervention with phytochemicals. Initiated cells may transform into precancerous cells spontaneously, but more commonly, tumor promoters such as chemicals or hormones stimulate the process. Chemoprotective agents may inactivate promoters, stimulate activity of protective enzyme machinery, or stabilize cell membranes to protect cell integrity. The phenolic and polyphenolic antioxidants are potent inhibitors of the promotion phase through a number of actions. Beta-carotene is considered to have its major effect at limiting the promotion phase in the development of cancer.[8, 9]

PROGRESSION

Progress of precancerous to cancerous cells involves further damage to the chromosomes and loss of cell regulation. This leads to uncontrolled growth of cells and tumor formation. Certain phytochemicals, such as soy isoflavones, decrease cell growth by limiting new blood vessel formation. Other phytochemicals may suppress tumor growth by enhancing immune surveillance and the ability of the immune system to limit formation of "foreign" cells. Selected phytochemicals may either inhibit the enzyme machinery necessary for cell growth (such as genistein inhibition of tyrosine kinase) or stimulate enzyme machinery that limits cell growth.[8]

The important role of the immune system in protection from cancer and in slowing of cancer cell growth cannot be covered here. One of the cutting-edge areas of cancer research is immunotherapy using antibodies developed to attack cancer cells. If our own immune system is operating well, we develop antibodies to nip new tumor growth in the bud. Antioxidants have an important role in ensuring that our immune system is fine-tuned and ready to attack any foreign tumor cells that may begin developing.[10]

PHYTOCHEMICALS ARE IMPORTANT IN CANCER PREVENTION

Table 4.1 lists some of the important phytochemicals, their food sources, and the types of cancers from which they may provide protection. Garlic and onions are rich in allyl sulfides, which serve to inactivate carcinogenic chemicals and promote their excretion from the body. Dried beans contain protease inhibitors, which slow down enzyme machinery required for tumor cell growth. Phytic acid binds iron and may prevent this potent oxidant from promoting free radical formation. Foods rich in beta-carotene may protect from cancer cell initiation or promotion as outlined above. Limonene from citrus fruits may stimulate production of enzymes that dispose of potential toxic chemicals. Cruciferous vegetables are rich in indoles, which stimulate enzymes that make estrogen less effective in promoting breast cancer, and isothiocyanates, which inactivate potential carcinogens before they can damage DNA.[11]

TABLE 4.1   SOME IMPORTANT PHYTOCHEMICALS THAT PROTECT FROM CANCER*

Food Source	Phytochemical	Cancer Protection[†]
Allium species (garlic, onion, etc.)	Organosulfur compounds	Intestines, stomach
Beans, dry	Protease inhibitors, phytic acid	Uncertain
Carrots, tomatoes, sweet potatoes, cantaloupe	Carotenoids[‡]	Breast, colon, esophagus, liver, lungs, mouth, stomach
Citrus fruit	Limonene, vitamin C[‡]	Esophagus, larynx, mouth, pancreas
Cruciferous vegetables (broccoli, cabbage, etc.)	Indoles, isothiocyanates	Bladder, cervix, colon, esophagus, larynx, lungs, mouth, ovary, pancreas, stomach
Fruit and vegetables	Many phytochemicals and antioxidants[‡]	Bladder, cervix, colon, esophagus, larynx, lungs, mouth, ovary, pancreas, stomach
Green tea	Many polyphenols[‡] (catechins)	Esophagus, lungs, stomach
Purple grapes, juice, red wine	Polyphenols[‡] (ellagic acid)	Uncertain
Soybeans	Isoflavones (genistein, daidzein)[‡]	Breast, prostate
Vegetables	Sulfurophane	Bladder, cervix, colon, esophagus, larynx, lungs, mouth, ovary, pancreas, stomach

* Modified from Boutwell.[27]
[†] Estimates from human studies and animal experiments.
[‡] These chemicals have important antioxidant properties.

Green tea contains a family of polyphenols, including the cate-chins, which may decrease risk for cancer of the esophagus, stom-ach, and lungs by protecting DNA.[12] Purple grapes and red wine are rich in polyphenols such as ellagic acid, which may protect from ini-tiation or promotion of tumor cells of various types.[9] Soybeans are unique sources of isoflavones such as genistein and daidzein, which have protective effects from breast and prostate cancer (see Chapter 7). Vegetables, of course, have a wide array of phytochemicals and antioxidants in addition to those specifically provided in cruciferous and carotenoid-rich species. Vegetable intake shows one of the strongest correlations with protection from cancer of any of the food groups.[13–16]

VEGETABLE AND FRUIT INTAKE PROTECT AGAINST CANCER

Fresh fruits and vegetables are generally rich in vitamins A, C, beta-carotene, and a wide variety of phytochemicals. Many studies indi-cate that eating more fresh fruits and vegetables significantly reduces risk of a number of different cancers.[11, 13–15] However, the individual or synergistic effects of antioxidants, phytochemicals, low fat intake, and high dietary fiber intake cannot be assessed. Use of single or combinations of phytochemicals may not be a magic bullet, and the intake of a variety of fruits and vegetables is important for health. Table 4.2 summarizes some of the major studies showing protective effects of vegetable and fruit intake on risk of various cancers. The authors of the review papers carefully assessed the strength of the scientific evidence and indicated a benefit only if the evidence was very strong.

TABLE 4.2   MAJOR STUDIES SHOWING THAT ANTIOXIDANT VITAMINS OR
VEGETABLES AND FRUITS HAVE PROTECTIVE EFFECTS FROM
DEVELOPMENT OF CANCER FOR HUMANS

AUTHOR (LOCATION)	FOOD OR NUTRIENT	CANCER PROTECTION*
Blot et al.[1] (China)	Beta-carotene, vitamin E, and selenium	All deaths from cancer Stomach
Mayne et al.[18] (New York State)	Beta-carotene, vitamin E, vegetables and fruits	Lung cancer (in nonsmokers)
Zaridze et al.[21] (Russia)	Beta-carotene	Colon
REVIEWS		
Block et al.[14]	Vegetables and fruits	Bladder, cervix, colon esophagus, larynx, lungs, mouth, ovary, pancreas, stomach
Byers and Perry[5]	Beta-carotene	Lungs, cervix
Byers and Perry[5]	Vitamin C	Pancreas, stomach
Flagg et al.[23]	Beta-carotene	Lungs, mouth
Flagg et al.[23]	Vitamin C	Mouth, cervix
Flagg et al.[23]	Vitamin E	Lungs
Steinmetz and Potter[13]	Vegetables and fruits	A variety of cancers
Zeigler[15]	Beta-carotene	Lungs

* These protective effects are reported to be statistically significant for humans.

Dr. Gladys Block and colleagues[14] reviewed almost two hundred different scientific studies. They reported that high intakes of fruits and vegetables were associated with a significant reduction in risk for cancer of the bladder, cervix, colon, esophagus, larynx, lung, mouth, ovary, pancreas, and stomach. In a similar extensive review, Steinmetz and Potter[13, 17] concluded that vegetable and fruit intake was associated with protection from all of the same cancers except for ovarian cancer. The study of Mayne and colleagues[18] also notes that vegetable and fruit intake is protective from lung cancer. All these authors conclude that eating a wide variety and generous amount of vegetables and fruits has a major protective effect from these cancers.

Unfortunately, intake of generous amounts of fruits and vegetables does not clearly protect from hormone-related cancers such as breast and prostate cancer. The strongest protection from these cancers appears to come from intake of soybeans and soy protein products rich in isoflavones.[19, 20] These benefits are discussed more fully in Chapter 7.

EATING SMART QUIZ

Are you eating smart? Take this quick, simple quiz by checking YES or NO to each question to find out how your diet compares to the American Cancer Society's nutrition guidelines. The guidelines are designed to help reduce your risk of cancer.

YES   NO

☐ ☐ 1. I rarely add butter or margarine to foods in cooking or at the table.

☐ ☐ 2. I rarely (less than twice a week) eat fried foods.

☐ ☐ 3. I drink only low-fat or skim milk and seldom eat high-fat cheeses such as jack, cheddar, Colby, Swiss, and cream cheese.

☐ ☐ 4. I seldom eat high-fat snack foods—potato or corn chips, nuts, buttered popcorn, and/or candy bars.

☐ ☐ 5. I take it easy on high-fat, baked goods such as pies, cakes, cookies, sweet rolls, and doughnuts.

☐ ☐ 6. I try to trim the fat from red meat and eat poultry without the skin.

☐ ☐ 7. I seldom eat bacon, hot dogs, ham, or luncheon meats.

☐ ☐ 8. I eat whole grain breads or pasta, brown rice, or whole grain cereal every day.

☐ ☐ 9. I eat foods rich in vitamin C—such as citrus fruits and juices, strawberries, tomatoes, and/or green peppers—every day.

☐ ☐ 10. I eat dark green and deep yellow fruits and vegetables often. (These include broccoli, greens, carrots, and peaches.)

☐ ☐ 11. I often eat vegetables of the cabbage family—broccoli, cabbage, cauliflower, or brussels sprouts.

☐ ☐ 12. I never, or only occasionally, drink alcohol.

HOW DO YOU RATE?

0-4 YES answers: Diet Alert
Your diet is probably too high in fat and too low in fiber-rich foods. You may want to take a look at your eating habits and find ways to make some changes. To start out, try adding more fruits and vegetables.

4-8 YES answers: Not Bad! You're Halfway There
You still have a way to go. Look at your NO answers to help you decide which areas of your diet need to be improved. Remember to cut down on high-fat foods and eat more fiber-rich foods such as whole grains and cereals.

9-12 YES answers: Good For You! You're Eating Smart
You should feel very good about yourself. You have been careful to limit your fats and eat a healthy diet. Keep up the good habits and keep looking for ways to improve.

For more information about diet and Eating Smart, contact your local American Cancer Society or call 1-800-ACS-2345.

ANTIOXIDANT VITAMINS PROTECT AGAINST CANCER

As summarized in the opening of this chapter, the intake of beta-carotene, vitamin E, and selenium supplements significantly reduced deaths from all types of cancer and from stomach cancer in a Chinese county.[1] Dr. Mayne and colleagues[18] reported that beta-carotene intake and vitamin E intake are associated with a significantly lower rate of lung cancer in nonsmokers (Table 4.2). Zaridze and colleagues[21] recently reported that beta-carotene intake protected from development of colon cancer.

Several experts have carefully reviewed the evidence linking antioxidant vitamins to protection from cancer (Table 4.2). These reviews indicate that beta-carotene protects from cancer of the lung and oral cavity and perhaps the cervix. Vitamin C protects from cancer of the mouth, pancreas, stomach, and perhaps cervix. Vitamin E reduces risk for lung cancer. The effects of the antioxidant vitamins on risk for these and other types of cancer are currently being assessed in a number of careful clinical studies.[5]

THE GREAT VITAMIN SCARES OF 1994 AND 1996

In April 1994 a Finnish research group reported results of a supplement trial in Finnish male smokers.[22] They followed more than twenty-nine thousand men for five to eight years. This study provided four treatments: placebo, a harmless capsule without vitamins; beta-carotene, 20 mg per day; vitamin E, 50 mg per day; and beta-carotene and vitamin E. The surprising outcome of this study is that men receiving beta-carotene developed lung cancer at a rate 18 percent higher than men on placebo.

Then, in January of 1996, the National Cancer Institute (NCI) terminated the use of beta-carotene and vitamin A in its Carotene and Retinol Efficacy Trial (CARET), a study designed to last six years to determine if a combination of the two substances could protect against lung cancer. The 18,314 people being studied were at high risk for cancer since all were long-term smokers or ex-smokers, and workers who had been exposed to cancer-causing asbestos. NCI ended the intervention portion of the CARET study 21 months before it was due to be completed because preliminary data indicated that the two substances "provide no benefit and may be causing harm." Furthermore, another clinical trial involving beta-carotene, the Physicians Health Study, had ended a few weeks earlier (December 31, 1995) without showing either significant positive or negative effects on the participants, 22,071 U.S. male physicians. In that trial, 22,071 doctors, 11% of whom were current smokers and 51% of whom had smoked at some time in their life, took either 50 mg of beta-carotene every other day or a placebo and 325 mg of aspirin or a placebo on the alternate day.

The fact that the results of the Physicians Health Study showed no benefits from beta-carotene was disappointing to researchers and millions of vitamin-takers alike, but at least that study showed no danger from the supplements. However, the declaration by NCI that beta-carotene supplements in the CARET "may be causing harm" was a bombshell. Newspapers throughout the country carried a January 19, 1996 Associated Press story inaccurately saying that NCI "researchers shut down a vitamin study of 18,000 smokers almost two years early because too many of those being given high doses of beta-carotene were dying." More evenhandedly, *The New York Times* reported that "one of the studies found that it (beta-carotene) *might even* be harmful to some people." Vitamin consumers were shocked and confused. Overreacting stockbrokers, fearing that Americans would stop taking vitamin supplements, advised their clients to sell the stock of companies, such as the General Nutrition store chain, that sell vitamins.

Actually, when the intervention phase of CARET was stopped, 974 participants had died from multiple causes, and 388 people had been diagnosed with lung cancer. A large majority of these deaths and lung cancer cases were expected. The smokers and former smokers had a smoking history of at least 20 "pack years," that is they smoked one pack per day for 20 years or two packs per day for 10 years. Still, the death rate among study participants was 17% higher and the lung cancer incidence was 28% higher than expected. Although these interim results were *not* statistically significant in a scientific sense, in light of the Finnish study the decision was made to tell the participants to stop taking beta-carotene and vitamin A. Researchers at the University of Washington School of Public Health, Seattle, will monitor the CARET participants for five more years to determine long-term effects of the beta-carotene intervention.

Dr. Jeffrey Blumberg, chief of the Antioxidants Research Laboratory at Tufts University, Boston, points out that the NCI announcement did not elaborate on the observation that former smokers, who comprised 34% of the CARET participants when recruited, appeared to respond more favorably to vitamin A and beta-carotene than current smokers, actually showing a 20% decrease in lung cancer risk! Furthermore, according to Dr. Blumberg, NCI sources seem to be blaming the adverse outcome of the 28% increase in lung cancer risk among all treated subjects on the beta-carotene supplements, despite the inability of the study to distinguish the effects of beta-carotene from the effects of the high dosage of vitamin A that was also given to participants. Many experts consider 25,000 IU of vitamin A to be a toxic dose.

It is important to appreciate that the beta-carotene results of the earlier Finnish study have been called into question because *all the excess lung cancer cases were found to be in a sub-population in the study who continued to smoke and to drink alcoholic beverages.* When the CARET data is fully analyzed, we believe a similar result may be found.

Also, due to the limitations associated with their design and intent, clinical trials may have limited relevance to issues of health promotion and disease prevention among the general population.

The idea that clinical trials such as these can give definitive answers is incorrect. Trials such as these are conducted in high-risk groups to shorten the length of time needed to see results, but the results may not be generalizable to healthy individuals. Because each clinical trial can test only a few substances at a time using a limited range of dosages, questions will always remain. Right now people are dying prematurely of heart disease and cancer. Do we really want to discourage use of supplements that have benefits that have been well documented? We don't think so.

We don't believe that the results cited in these two studies will stand the test of time. For one thing, the amounts of beta-carotene may have been too large. The 30 mg dose of beta-carotene in CARET is equivalent to about two medium-sized carrots. Also the participants in that study were getting another 25,000 IU of vitamin A. The supplemental beta-carotene Dr. Anderson recommends is equivalent to less than one carrot daily.

It should also be pointed out that the CARET and Physicians Health Study trials didn't investigate the other potentially beneficial effects of supplementary beta-carotene, particularly the benefits that occur when this substance is taken together with other substances such as aspirin and nutrients such as vitamins C and E. The aspirin component of the Physicians Health Study was dropped several years ago after aspirin was shown to be effective. While the data at the time showed the combination of aspirin and beta-carotene to be even more effective than either one alone, that data was not cited during the NCI announcement.

We now know that there is a synergistic interrelationship between the antioxidants, that they work more effectively together than when taken alone. We are not worried about the safety of vitamins C, E, or beta-carotene since they have been components of foods for millennia. The amounts of beta-carotene we recommend as supplements are readily available in the diet. No one is recommending that people avoid carrots, sweet potatoes and cantaloupe.

Indeed, immediately after the NCI announcement, the American Cancer Society (ACS) represented by Michael Thun, M.D., director of Analytic Epidemiology for that organization, stated: "While a recently released study casts doubt on the role beta-carotene, as a dietary supplement, plays in cancer prevention, there is strong scientific evidence that diets high in fruits and vegetables, a source of many natural nutrients in addition to beta-carotene, are associated with lower risk of many forms of cancer."

These disappointing studies need to be put in perspective. As summarized in Tables 4.1 and 4.2, there is extensive evidence that intake of beta-carotene or vegetables rich in beta-carotene is associated with lower risk for several types of cancer. In fact, ten separate reports indicate that high levels of beta-carotene are associated with lower risk for several types of cancer, including lung cancer. The Chinese study summarized at the beginning of this chapter found that beta-carotene, when combined with vitamin E and selenium, reduced deaths from all forms of cancer by 13 percent;[1] in this same study, risk for lung cancer was reduced by 45 percent.[2] So the observations of the Finnish researchers cannot currently be explained, but this represents a minority report. Most experts feel that beta-carotene protects from development of lung cancer and other forms of cancer.[5, 15, 23]

TO SUPPLEMENT OR NOT TO SUPPLEMENT?

Use of antioxidant supplements, especially beta-carotene, remains controversial. However, there is no controversy about the value of a diet that emphasizes generous amounts of fruits and vegetables, rich sources of many nutrients that protect against a variety of cancers. Most of the laboratory studies indicate that antioxidants have an important role in blocking or decreasing the initiation and/or promotion stages of development of experimental cancers; antioxidants may also decrease progression of tumors by strengthening the immune system. Many studies indicate that the antioxidant vitamins, given as supplements, decrease risk of certain types of cancer. The risks against taking antioxidant supplements at the doses commonly recommended (and at the doses we recommend in Table 8.1) are very small. So why shouldn't everyone take antioxidant supplements?

The arguments against taking antioxidant supplements are as follows:

- Taking supplements may diminish commitment to other healthy behaviors, such as not smoking or eating vegetables and fruits;
- Much of the health-promoting benefits of vegetables and fruits may reside in other phytochemicals or even natural antioxidants, and the supplements may not provide all of this specific protection;
- Supplements may have minor or annoying side effects, such as yellowing of the skin or stomach irritation;
- Taking a "full strength" antioxidant supplement may add unnecessary expense to one's budget.

After carefully considering all these factors, we strongly feel that the enormous potential health benefits from taking antioxidant supplements far outweigh the negative aspects and cautions. Of course, our antioxidant program includes a generous intake of vegetables and fruits, including the specific vegetables and fruits that are especially rich in antioxidants. So we encourage you to join us in this health-promoting behavior.

TO SUM UP

- Research studies, such as the recent one from China, indicate that intake of antioxidant supplements reduces total death rates from cancer.
- Fruits and vegetables are rich in many phytochemicals that have antioxidant and other health-promoting properties.
- Studies with experimental cancers indicate that antioxidants

and certain other phytochemicals decrease the conversion of normal cells into cancer-forming cells.

- Phytochemicals such as those from garlic, carrots, oranges, broccoli, green tea, red wine, soybeans, and vegetables act specifically to protect from certain types of cancer.
- Intake of generous amounts of vegetables and fruits protects from these cancers: bladder, cervix, colon, esophagus, larynx, lung, mouth, ovary, pancreas, and stomach.
- Intake of these antioxidants appears to protect from specific cancers: beta-carotene—lung, mouth, and perhaps cervix; vitamin C—pancreas and stomach; and vitamin E—lung.

WHAT YOU CAN DO

GENERAL PREVENTION

If you are in good health and do not have a strong family tendency toward cancer, you still want to reduce your risk of developing cancer.

- Have regular physical examinations, blood tests, and mammograms as recommended by your doctor.
- Begin the antioxidant diet and exercise program outlined in the left-hand column in Table 8.1. Having five servings of vegetables and fruits and one can of vegetable juice daily give you specific protection from cancer.
- Start taking one multivitamin-mineral capsule, two antioxidant capsules, and one enteric-coated aspirin per day.
- Begin addressing the health-promoting behaviors listed in Table 8.1 under the column labeled "Other."

TAILORED PROTECTION AND DISEASE REVERSAL

If you have a strong family history of cancer (e.g., a parent, aunt or uncle, or sibling with breast or colon cancer), you will want to begin the antioxidant program as soon as possible to reduce your risk of cancer. If you have had a diagnosis of some type of cancer (other than skin cancer) you probably are already doing most of these things. The list on page 70 will serve as a checklist to ensure that you are on the full antioxidant program.

JIM'S DIARY

In October 1995 I had the opportunity to spend two weeks in China. I was invited to present a lecture on soy protein and blood cholesterol at an international nutrition conference focusing on health problems of Asian people. The focus of the conference was on nutrition to reduce risk for heart disease, cancer, and other health problems. Obesity is increasing rapidly in China, as they now eat much more fat than previously. Vegetable consumption is on the decline as more people move to cities. Heart disease and certain forms of cancer are expected to increase as people increase their fat intake. Two major protectors remaining in the diet are green or black tea and tofu. I learned to prepare green tea in my hotel room, to enjoy it first thing in the morning and later in the day, and to have it with meals. I purchased a pound of green tea, and my wife, Gay, and I enjoy it each morning. I add one tablespoon of green tea leaves in a medium-size (one quart) teapot and fill it with boiling water. After it brews for ten minutes, we strain it into cups and into a thermos for later use. The remaining tea from the morning is used as iced tea at night.

I also enjoyed many different forms of tofu in China. I traveled with a group including one vegetarian from California. She ordered tofu at every meal and shared the tofu with me. In this book we include several tofu recipes for you to try. Now I have tofu at least three times per week. Instead of going to a cafeteria for vegetables on Sunday, we now often have lunch at a Chinese restaurant, where I can order tofu.

5

PRESERVE BRAIN FUNCTION AND PREVENT DETERIORATION

LINDA'S GREATEST FEAR IS REALIZED: SHE DEVELOPS THE TYPE OF MEMORY LOSS HER MOTHER HAD

Linda is sixty-five years old. She has played many roles: a wonderful wife, mother, friend, neighbor, relative, and church member. Unfortunately, for the past five years she has experienced bothersome memory problems. She can remember the distant past quite well but doesn't remember what she heard a few minutes ago. Her husband, Paul, is very supportive, but sometimes gets impatient with his wife's memory lapses. He often feels depressed. No wonder. Paul had retired early, and they had planned to travel. Now, however, Linda feels comfortable only at home. She seldom leaves it, even to spend the night at her sister's house. She clings to familiar surroundings and to her daily routine.

Linda's mother had been a brilliant woman. She completed her college bachelor's degree at an early age and taught for many years. She earned a Ph.D. at age sixty and had self-sufficiently lived alone until she died at age eighty-eight. However, during the last eighteen years of her life she was bothered by short-term memory lapses.

One of Linda's greatest fears was that she would develop memory problems like her mother. Unfortunately, Linda's fears seem to be coming true—she seems to be developing the same type of memory problems her mother had. Even before Linda started staying home all the time, she often misplaced her car keys and often forgot the names of new people she had met, even after encountering them several times. At home she often found herself standing before an open pantry or open refrigerator door, forgetting what she had wanted to get.

Like their father, Linda's son and daughter are devoted to their mother. They are frustrated by her memory problems and are very worried that they may also develop this apparently inherited form of early memory loss. Linda has been extensively evaluated medically and does not have a classical form of Alzheimer's disease, but she does have a form of dementia (loss of brain function) that closely resembles her mother's problem.

In light of our current knowledge about antioxidants and their protective role, Dr. Anderson advised Linda's children to follow our active tailored protection program (see Chapter 8) to reduce their risks for developing memory loss as they get older. Linda is also on the program. Although we can't claim dramatic improvement in her condition, Paul is convinced that not only has the rate of her short-term memory loss been slowed but also that Linda even has a slightly improved memory in that she doesn't forget where she put things as much.

SLOW THE LOSS OF BRAIN CELLS

One of the major fears of aging is that we will be disabled and be a burden to our families. Most of us want to live a long life but avoid the loss of mental function such as memory. To retain full mental capabilities into our later years, we have to do two things:

1. assure our brains a generous intake of antioxidants;
2. use our minds as much as possible.

Brain cells are unlike many other cells in the body. They cannot reproduce themselves after we reach adulthood. In terms of absolute numbers, our brain cells "max out" (to use the words of our teenage sons) at about age nineteen. By early adulthood we actually start losing brain cells. Luckily, our brains have trillions of cells to spare. It is said that Einstein used only 11 percent of his brain. Most people use even smaller percentages. Unused brain cells represent untapped potential. We can learn to tap that potential by putting our brains into training. Just as we exercise our bodies, we also have to exercise our brains. We will soon explain how to do just that, but right now let's concentrate on learning how to slow brain cell loss.

Recent research indicates that free radicals contribute to loss of brain cells during normal aging and in diseases such as Alzheimer's and Parkinson's. New laboratory techniques have been used to demonstrate that the protein in the brains of elderly people and in the brains of Alzheimer's sufferers has been oxidized by free radical damage. Medical researchers had long thought that "oxidative stress"[1] caused damage to brain cells and led to deficiencies in thinking ability and memory as we age. Now these researchers have evidence that this is so.

Oxidative stress occurs when free radicals overwhelm the brain's antioxidant defenses. As we have seen in previous chapters, normally free radicals and the processes generating them are kept in check or neutralized by antioxidant defense mechanisms. However, as we get older our brains face a twofold problem. First, because of decreased brain blood supply, the number of free radicals attacking our brain cells increases. Second, our defense systems—naturally occurring brain antioxidants—decrease because of cell loss during aging. Many scientific studies have shown that lower amounts of brain antioxidants, especially deficiencies of vitamin E, are caused by "a decrease in the antioxidant defense systems of the brain."[2]

Even though the brain's naturally occurring antioxidant defenses become depleted as we age, impairment during one's senior years is not inevitable. Scientific evidence shows that we can bolster the brain's natural antioxidant defenses with vitamins E and C, both of which "aid in protecting the brain from oxidative stress by directly scavenging toxic radicals."[3] That's why we need to deliver more antioxidants to our brains. Remember, the normal American diet doesn't supply enough vitamin E and other antioxidants, so the problem remains how to get the antioxidant protectors to the battlefield—to the brain.

THE BRAIN: A BATTLEFIELD WITH WEAK DEFENSES AGAINST FREE RADICAL ATTACKS

Free radicals do more damage to the brain than to any other part of the body.[4] The brain is extremely vulnerable to free radical oxidation for several reasons. First, it uses large amounts of oxygen and is thus exposed to hordes of free radicals. Although the brain constitutes only 2 percent of body weight, in a resting individual it consumes a whopping 20 percent of the body's oxygen, and even more when a person is exercising. Second, one-tenth of the brain is composed of lipids,[5] fat molecules made up of readily oxidizable polyunsaturated fatty acids.[6] The membranes of our nerves, neurons, and other brain cells are made up of trillions of these fat molecules, so free radicals have plenty of targets to attack. Proportionately speaking, ten times the number of free radicals attack the brain than any other organ. It is no wonder that every day we lose so many brain cells.

If we lose so many brain cells daily, why are not more of us victims of neurological diseases? First, the brain is a miracle of creation. It is composed of so many cells that there are backups for almost every cell function that is lost to free radical damage. For most people, it is only after years of constant free radical attack that thought and memory processes begin to fail.

Let's now learn about some of the most feared brain and nervous system diseases and how their onset might be delayed or prevented by the use of antioxidants.

ALZHEIMER'S DISEASE

Alzheimer's is one of the most common chronic diseases of older persons. More than 10 percent of persons over age sixty-five suffer from this condition. In addition, a large number of seniors have other forms of dementia that impair mental functions such as memory or planning and thus interfere with the enjoyment of life.[7]

Alzheimer's disease brings loss of memory, impaired judgment, and emotional instability. Different people have different types of losses. Linda, like her mother, mainly suffered from memory loss, but for the most part retained emotional stability.

A form of dementia referred to as "an age-related torpor of the senses, and stupefaction of the intellectual functions"[8] was described by Aretaeus of Cappadocia in the second century A.D. However, it was only at the beginning of the twentieth century that Dr. Alois Alzheimer, a Bavarian psychiatrist, identified the specific pathogenic changes that the disease that now bears his name causes in the human brain. Now, almost ninety years after Dr. Alzheimer first described the buildup of plaque and tangled neurofibers that characterize this disease, we know at least one factor behind their cause: "The nerve cell degeneration of Alzheimer's disease is exactly what we would expect from the action of free radicals," said Dr. J. Steven Richardson at an Alzheimer's Association-sponsored medical research meeting.[9]

By autopsying the brains of deceased Alzheimer's disease patients, medical researchers have discovered that the disease damages the axons and dendrites of the brain. The damage apparently involves a protein fragment called amyloid protein. When excessive buildups of amyloid protein accumulate, it clogs and tangles the brain's neural network, disrupting normal functions. The buildup of these senile plaques occur within the cerebral cortex, hippocampus, amygdala, and other brain areas, all vital to the process of thought and memory.

According to one theory, amyloid protein causes Alzheimer's disease because it chokes off and causes brain neurons to die. But what causes amyloid proteins to form plaque? Scientists don't know for sure. They know that amyloid protein in a "mature" plaque, one that has taken years, even decades to form, is "chemically modified as compared with that found in blood vessels."[10] Could that chemical change be sparked by oxidation? Some researchers feel that Alzheimer's disease has a specific genetic component. Researchers, however, have been unable to find a specific defect in the genes of patients with the disease. This led them to the conclusion that Alzheimer's disease is caused by "many different genetic defects on different chromosomes."[11] But what could these defects have in common? Could it be a genetic mutation caused by oxidation? Research is being done that may answer these questions.

As medical knowledge has increased, physicians have identified several related dementias they now call dementias of the Alzheimer type (DAT). "Several vitamins possess a potential for therapeutic use in DAT due to their direct interaction with the (free) radical mechanism. Most important are alpha-tocopherol (vitamin E), ascorbic acid (vitamin C), and retinoic acid (vitamin A)," states a recent report in the medical journal *Drug Research*.[12] The report cites many studies that have linked the development of Alzheimer's disease to the intake of aluminum found in certain foods and water. Although most authorities believe that such studies remain inconclusive, experts from three other countries (England, Japan, and Switzerland), writing in a prestigious medical journal, state that "limiting the intake of aluminum . . . *and the use of antioxidant micronutrient supplements* and drugs provides a rational and feasible therapeutic strategy."[13]

PARKINSON'S DISEASE

First described by the English physician Dr. James Parkinson, the disease that bears his name is a slowly progressive, degenerative disorder of the central nervous system that causes muscular rigidity, slowness of movement, tremor, and postural instability. It is the fourth most common neurodegenerative disease of the elderly, affecting about 1 percent of the population over age sixty-five.

We previously mentioned studies that indicate that oxidative stress involving the burning of fats contributes to the development of Parkinson's disease (PD). Researchers believe that this oxidant stress is a major factor leading to degeneration of brain and motor neurons in PD patients. "When free radical generation exceeds the capacity of antioxidant defenses, the result is oxidative stress," which contributes to the development of Parkinson's disease, writes Japanese medical school professor Toshikazu Yoshikawa.[14] Several other studies have found that PD sufferers have elevated oxidative damage of the fatty tissues of their brains, particularly in the *substantia nigra* section of the midbrain. Microscopic examination of this area of the brain reveals loss of neurons.[15] "Polyunsaturated fatty acids and glutathione (a free radical-fighting antioxidant) was decreased," according to still another study.[16]

This research leads scientists to strongly believe that treatment with antioxidants can help patients in the early stages of Parkinson's disease. Indeed, a preliminary study shows that antioxidant therapy slowed the progression of Parkinson's disease. A cohort of early-stage PD patients taking vitamins C and E were compared to a similar group not taking the antioxidants. Those not taking antioxidants were forced to take the anti-Parkinson's drug L-dopa (levodopa) 2½ years before the antioxidant-taking group.

VITAMIN E THERAPY FOR PARKINSON'S DISEASE

Vitamin E is the major fat-soluble, chain-breaking antioxidant that protects cell membranes. It specifically protects cell membrane polyunsaturated fatty acids (PUFAs) from lipid perioxidation—that is, the oxidation or burning up of the fat cells.[17] Studies indicate that vitamin E treatment in patients with early, untreated Parkinson's disease delays the time required before patients are forced to take drugs such as levodopa to control the condition.[18] "Beginning in 1979 I suggested to all patients with early PD who were not yet receiving levodopa therapy that it would be reasonable for them to take high dosages of alpha-tocopherol (vitamin E) and ascorbate (vitamin C)," wrote Columbia University neurologist Stanley Fahn in a 1992 article in *Annals of Neurology*. He conducted a pilot study of seventy-two patients with early PD and compared the time it became necessary for the treated patients to take levadopa to another group of patients who did not receive antioxidants. "The time when levodopa became necessary was extended by 2½ years in the group receiving alpha-tocopherol and ascorbate. Results of this study suggest that the PD's progression may be slowed by administration of those oxidants."[19] Dr. Fahn called for further large-scale studies to be carried out. Indeed, a group of researchers known as the Parkinson Study Group is involved in a clinical trial of hundreds of early-stage Parkinson's disease patients using the drug deprenyl and tocopherol, the component of vitamin E that traps free radicals. The ongoing study uses the double-blind method, which means that neither the investigators nor the patients know which patients are receiving vitamin E, which are receiving the drug, and which are receiving a combination of the two. Results won't be known until the study ends.

USE IT OR LOSE IT—CALISTHENICS TO KEEP YOUR MIND IN SHAPE

One of the myths of aging is that belief that as you grow older your mind steadily deteriorates until you manifest symptoms of senility or a progressive dementia such as Alzheimer's disease. That's just not true. The brain works much like a muscle—given the proper amount of rest, the harder you use it, the healthier it gets. While it's true that every decade we lose about 10 percent of our neurons, the brain cells that control higher thought, we don't necessarily lose the capacity to think, remember, or learn.

One reason we can still function cognitively is that our brains are full of redundant neurons and the circuitry that connects them. Another reason is that the brain is quite clever in making connections between its own neurons. Have you ever formatted a computer disk to make it ready to accept data from a computer? Figuratively speaking, your mind is constantly laying down information-carrying grooves in your brain, like a computer establishes information-carrying tracks on a blank floppy disk. When stimulated by work or play, brain neurons rapidly sprout new connections between each other. Those connections are ultrathin neurofibers called axons and dendrites. Axons are the outgoing message carriers and dendrites are the receivers of messages from other cells. These connections and the rate at which they are made, not the nerve cells themselves, determine how well we think and remember.

The rate at which axon and dendrite connections are made depends on how often we intellectually challenge ourselves. No matter how old you are, the more you stimulate your brain, the more you can stimulate the growth of interconnected axons and dendrites. As you increase those interconnections, you also increase your odds of preventing or reversing degenerative damage to the brain.

People who keep their brains stimulated with interesting work, higher education, or even interesting leisure activities not only keep themselves mentally sharp, they even receive protection against the debilitation of Alzheimer's disease and other dementias, according to an intriguing article in the prestigious *Journal of the American Medical Association* titled "Influence of Education and Occupation on the Incidence of Alzheimer's Disease." The researchers' data indicate that "increased education and occupational attainment may reduce the risk of Alzheimer's."[20] The important thing is to consistently expose yourself to mental challenges. "Anything that is intellectually challenging can probably serve as a kind of stimulus for axon and dendritic growth, which means it helps protect the mental fitness of your brain."[21]

As exercise physiologists say, "use it or lose it." In a moment we will recommend a series of mental calisthenics that use your physical senses such as sight, hearing, smell, taste, and touch. A husband-wife team of experts in the field of neuropsychology confirms that these exercises enhance brain power. "After all," states psychologist Miriam Ehrenberg, coauthor of the book *Optimum Brain Power,* "information about the world comes to us through our senses and this information serves as a foundation for our intelligence." Her coauthor and husband, Dr. Otto Ehrenberg, also a psychologist, adds: "One of the most important principles in being more intelligent is to drink up as much information as you can. Acquiring information builds neural pathways that expand your brain's capacity."[22]

Exercise experts remind us that exercise not only makes us fitter, it also makes us smarter. "There are many studies in the medical and psychological literature which show that people who exercise on a regular basis[24] are more apt to be mentally fit," says Dr. Raymond Harris, author of the popular book *Fitness After 50*. "Insufficient oxygen to cerebral nerve cells leads to a die-off of certain neurotransmitters and diminished brain function. As a person becomes more physically fit with exercise, the general circulation improves allowing more oxygen-carrying blood to flow to the brain. Increased blood flow to the brain is one of the factors behind the improved mental abilities noted in these studies."[25]

Here are our suggested mental calisthenics, developed with the help of many experts, including the Ehrenbergs:[23]

• Use your eyes. We are used to focusing on one object or person within our visual field. Exercise: Take a moment or two to be conscious of the "big picture," taking in everything in your visual field. Then shift your focus from object to object, or especially if you're with other people, from person to person. If you look too long at any one person or thing, you stop really seeing it, points out Dr. Miriam Ehrenberg.

• Use your ears. Don't be a passive or careless listener. Too often schools or colleges have conditioned us to listen passively to teachers and lecturers. As a result, we often get tranquilized rather than stimulated. Be an active listener by consciously thinking of whether you agree with or even understand the speaker. Interrupt, if possible, to ask questions or discuss a particular point. The speaker's point is more apt to stick with you if you ask questions. Exercise. For one minute daily, stop what you are doing, close your eyes, and just listen to the sounds around you. You will probably be amazed or at least surprised at what you hear that ordinarily you are oblivious to. Things you might notice include traffic noises, a dog barking, a bird singing, the sound of car tires on the road, or the automatic switching on or off of your air conditioner or heater. Especially try this exercise when you are in new surroundings.

• Use your nose. As adults our sense of smell is poorly used, but realize that your nose can tell you a lot that other senses cannot because smell lingers. Children, who have more sensitive senses of smell than adults, often can tell who visited the home while they were in school, identifying visitors by the perfume or after-shave odor. Exercise: Take a minute each day to concentrate on the smells in your surroundings. Walk around the room you are in and sniff. Try to identify individual smells. For instance, is that the aroma of coffee or tea coming from the kitchen? Can you smell what your neighbor is cooking? On the next day, change your surroundings when you do this exercise. Try it outdoors as well as indoors.

• Use your sense of taste. Too many of us gulp our food without enjoying it. Several minutes of concentrated tasting every day will activate unused taste buds and unused brain neurons, forging new connections between the taste buds and the brain. Exercise: Select a piece of fruit or a crunchy raw vegetable and bite into it. Don't hurry. Savor it. Pay attention to its texture and taste. Allow your taste buds to revel in its full flavor. Close your eyes when you are chewing, and do nothing with your hands. Allow nothing to distract you as you focus your thoughts on the taste of the food in your mouth. Pay close attention to the sensations as the food caresses your tongue and slides from your mouth and down your throat on its way to your stomach. Now repeat with another small bite. Close your eyes. Savor the taste. The important part of this exercise is to focus your attention on the internal sensations that occur when you eat. This exercise not only builds brain neurons and allows you to enjoy food more, but also if you practice a longer version of this exercise during meals, it can help you cut down on the amount of food you eat because you'll get more satisfaction from less food and will fill up faster.

• Use your sense of touch. Do you realize that our sense of touch can be separated into various components? For instance, we can feel temperature, whether something is hot or cold. We can also feel pressure, changes in intensity, and the position of various objects. Exercise: To develop your sensitivity to touch, spend at least sixty seconds daily feeling some object. Choose a different object or several objects each day, but spend at least sixty seconds with each. With your eyes closed, concentrate on your tactile sensations. Pass the object from one hand to another. Feel all sides of the object, tracing your fingers over its entire surface, feeling its contours and crevices. Notice the feeling of the object on your skin. How would you describe it to others? Is it smooth, rough, fuzzy, or does it tingle?

OTHER WAYS TO STIMULATE YOUR BRAIN

• Play games. Any activity involving fine movement also develops coordination and creates new connections between brain neurons. Ping-Pong, squash, and racquetball are examples of vigorous games. Less vigorous games include building card houses or playing pick-up-sticks with a child. You can also work crossword puzzles and do anagrams on your own, or play other word games with your spouse, children, or friends.

• Work with your hands. Working with beads to create elaborate designs or doing various types of needlework such as needlepoint or cross-stitching are effective exercises for the brain.

• Use your less favored hand for tasks. For instance, if you are right-handed, practice dialing the phone, undoing a knot, threading a needle, or writing with your left hand.

• Turn to the arts. Learn to paint or play a musical instrument. If you already play one, pick a different type. For instance, if you are a string player, try one of the horns. Albert Einstein played a violin. Winston Churchill painted landscapes.

SUMMARY

• The brain is composed of cells very vulnerable to oxidative damage, yet has relatively low levels of naturally occurring protective antioxidants. Since the brain uses one-fifth of the body's total oxygen, it is under heavy free radical attack.

• During an individual life span, millions of brain cells are lost to these free radical attacks. However, the brain, a masterwork of creation, is composed of trillions of cells, providing backup systems that enable most of us to function quite well mentally in our later years. It is only when these backup systems are overwhelmed by free radicals that people manifest cognitive and memory problems. Antioxidants act as "reinforcements," bolstering the brain's natural defenses.

• Alzheimer's disease is one of the most common and feared chronic brain diseases of the elderly. Preliminary studies indicate that antioxidants, especially vitamin E, may offer protection against early onset of this disease.

• Parkinson's disease is a slowly progressive disorder of the central nervous system. Preliminary research indicates that vitamin E therapy may delay, by up to 2½ years in early-stage Parkinson's disease patients, the time when symptoms become so severe that the patients have to take the drug levodopa. This is important to these patients because the beneficial effects of levodopa ultimately wear off and, as this book goes to press, the FDA has approved no drug to replace it. Thus, to Parkinson's disease patients who respond positively, vitamin E prolongs their productive lives.

• Mental calisthenics, especially those using your five senses— sight, hearing, smell, taste, and touch—can help keep your mind in shape.

86

WHAT YOU CAN DO NOW

- In Chapter 8 we explain the food portion of the antioxidant, antiaging program. Follow the advice in that chapter to delay, possibly prevent, or even reverse the adverse changes that normally occur in the brain with advancing age.
- Especially make sure you eat the recommended amounts of antioxidant-rich fruits and vegetables listed in that chapter.
- Don't forget to take your antioxidant supplements, especially the recommended amounts of vitamins C and E listed in Table 8.1.
- Exercise your mind. Remember, if you don't use it, you may lose it. Do the mental calisthenics and play the mind games listed above.

6

PREVENT OR DELAY THE ONSET OF AGING SKIN, ARTHRITIS, DIABETES, AND EYE DISEASES

"Every man desires to live long, but no man would be old" is a quote attributed to eighteenth-century Anglo-Irish poet Jonathan Swift. Although his choice of the words "every man" and "no man" is what we now would classify as male-chauvinistic, his main point stands true today for women as well as men. We would much rather be like "the wonderful one-hoss shay" in Oliver Wendell Holmes's poem "The Deacon's Masterpiece," which was built in "such a logical way" that it ran a hundred years in perfect working order and then painlessly crumbled away.

Unfortunately, we aren't like that wonderful contraption. As we get older we become more susceptible to degenerative processes associated with aging. Our skin dries up and wrinkles. We experience various aches, pains, and inflammations. Various internal organs and bodily process don't work as well as they did when we were younger. We tire faster than we did in the past.

These unpleasing but normal changes commonly associated with getting older are not only uncomfortable, they also set us up for even more serious diseases and disabilities associated with aging. If we could delay the onset of disability and degenerative disease we would not only add years to our lives but also add life to those years.

There is a connecting thread between many of the health problems associated with accelerated aging. Conditions as diverse as aging skin, arthritis, diabetes, and vision problems all share one attribute: They result from years of accumulated free radical trauma at the cellular level. Although many of the unpleasant changes wrought by aging are inevitable, how old you will be when they occur is variable.

Why do some people start to fall apart at age fifty or sixty, while others appear to resist the ravages of age in their seventies and older? Your genetic heritage plays a role, but it is just one factor. Aging is a multifactorial process. How you care for yourself physically, mentally, and nutritionally makes a difference. You might have a friend who has a wonderful genetic inheritance: His ancestors all lived to be a hundred. However, you'll probably outlive him if you follow the antioxidant, antiaging program while he abuses his body by smoking, overeating, and failing to exercise.

Perhaps you didn't treat your body as well in the past as you now wish you had. Even if you are experiencing adverse symptoms as a result of that early abuse, you can still benefit from going on our program. It's never too late to adopt health-promoting behaviors. If you are now experiencing symptoms associated with premature aging, consider them to be an alert signal, like the wake-up ring of your alarm clock. You may not be able to set the clock back, but you can keep it ticking. In other words, the antioxidant, antiaging program won't make you young again, but it can relieve the symptoms and in some cases actually reverse some of the cellular damage that has been done. Thus it is *not* inevitable that you have to succumb by inches to the degenerative conditions of aging. New information and insights about the importance of antioxidants and phytochemicals and the benefits of high fiber, combined with what we now know about the value of antioxidant/phytochemical supplementation (see Chapters 8 and 9) and the benefits of exercise (see Chapter 10), can make a life-extending healthy difference in your life. Our antioxidant, antiaging program may not make you younger, but it can make you feel younger and even live longer by delaying the onset of degenerative diseases and lessening the severity of the inevitable changes associated with getting older.

Let's now examine some of the common problems often experienced as people get older.

AGING SKIN

WHAT YOU NEED TO KNOW ABOUT YOUR SKIN

Although our skin is our body's largest organ, it replaces itself every twenty-eight days as old skin cells die and flake off and as new skin cells replace them. This constant cell replacement is necessary because the skin, our body's protective suit, is the first layer of defense against destructive outside forces such as ultraviolet (UV) light from the sun. The skin's job, according to dermatologist Joseph P. Bark, is to "prevent the portable sea that is our tissues, fluid, and blood from evaporating."[1] To accomplish this mission the skin has, over aeons, developed evaporative and convective cooling mechanisms that allow it to keep our innards within a relatively narrow, life-sustaining temperature band.

Yet too much exposure to the sun can threaten that balance by causing sunburn, a form of oxidization that in severe forms can interfere with the skin's cooling mechanisms. The UV light component of sunlight not only causes skin cancer but also encourages the creation of unstable oxygen molecules called free radicals, which are responsible for signs of premature skin aging such as wrinkling and the brown skin blotches called "liver spots." ("Liver spots" have nothing to do with the liver. As just pointed out, they have more to do with accelerated aging caused by long-term exposure to the UV component of sunlight.)

Unabsorbed free radicals can also cause undesirable, rusty cross-linkages between the protein chains that make up our skin. Protein chains are necessary for the skin to maintain elasticity and strength. When the protein chains of the skin are attacked by free radicals, they literally "rust" and twist together, losing their elasticity. Forehead wrinkles and "crow's-feet" are signs of free radical damage.

PREVENTION AND REPAIR OF SKIN DAMAGE

Antioxidant nutrients, especially vitamin E, are like an oilcan for the Tin Man, protecting the protein chains from rusting. Several studies have shown that the antioxidant vitamin E applied topically to the skin protects against free radicals and promotes healing. In one experiment, Dr. Barbara Gilchrest, a dermatologist at Boston University School of Medicine, exposed human cells in a test tube to UV light. She discovered that cells pretreated with vitamin E were more likely to survive than cells in the controlled environment without vitamin E. Other studies indicate that vitamin E has anti-inflammatory effects, promotes wound healing, and may even be "of clinical value in modifying undesirable scar formation."[2]

As a result of such research, many cosmetic companies now add vitamin E and other antioxidants to lotions, sunscreens, and other beauty products. Critics claim that combining vitamin E with other antioxidants is just a marketing gimmick and that not enough antioxidants are being added to make a difference. The critics raise a valid point. Research regarding moisturizing creams and other beauty products is lacking. However, there is evidence that small amounts of vitamin E can be a useful ingredient in sunscreens. Because of its ability to soak up free radicals, vitamin E can boost the effectiveness of sunscreens by several points on the sun prevention factor (SPF) scale.

Antioxidant supplementation, especially with vitamin E, can protect the skin against damage from the sun, affirms Dr. Ingrid Emerit, a leading French expert. "The majority of free radicals is formed as a consequence of light exposure . . . in addition [to other] defense systems, skin is protected by antioxidants. . . . Animal studies have shown that dietary antioxidant supplementation can result in marked reduction of number and severity of UV-induced carcinomas."[3] Among those animal studies are those at the University of Arizona. Scientists there found that more than two-thirds of the lab animals (mice) exposed to UV radiation developed skin cancer within thirty-one weeks. Reduced cancer rates were found when the diets of another group of the animals were supplemented with vitamin E.

Dr. Emerit believes that both oral intake and topical application of antioxidants in sunblockers can "diminish UV-induced free radical tissue injury" and offer long-term protection against UV if used regularly and *before* exposure to the sun. She warns that by age fifteen most Caucasians already have some deteriorations of the elastic fibers in their skin so "antioxidant administration has to start early. It should be pursued throughout the year, since even small fluctuations of UV light may generate free radicals. . . . Also, most antioxidants appear to be more protective before than after exposure to UV irradiation. Only regular use can therefore provide optimal conditions for protection."[4]

Dr. Emerit pointed out that studies have shown that vitamin E applied topically (on the surface of the skin) actually penetrates through the pores, hair follicles, and stratum corneum, the upper layer of the outer part of our skin. Four hours after administration, vitamin E still remains in those upper layers of the skin, according to one study using radioactive tracers. The same study revealed that vitamin E penetrated to the lower layers of the outer skin within twenty-four hours.

ARTHRITIS

WHAT YOU NEED TO KNOW ABOUT ARTHRITIS[5]

Inflammation, pain, tenderness, stiffness, swollen joints, and a decrease in mobility are just a few of the many symptoms that occur in the many forms of arthritis. Among the most common type of arthritis are:

• Rheumatoid, a chronic disease in which joints become stiff, painful, and inflamed. The inflammation can spread to other joints and ultimately can become crippling. It is believed to be caused by an immune reaction, possibly sparked by free radicals, against the joint tissues. An immune reaction occurs when a person's own immune system go to war against its own body.

• Ankylosing spondylitis, a chronic, progressive affliction that causes stiffening of the joints of the spine, so it is also commonly called spinal arthritis. This form of arthritis has been found in the spines of Egyptian mummies dating to 8000 B.C.

• Osteoarthritis, also known as degenerative joint disease. (Joints are the mechanisms that, when they work properly, allow for relatively friction-free motion between bones.) Osteoarthritis is a chronic inflammation of bones and joints due to degenerative changes in cartilage. The condition occurs mainly in the hips and knees of older people.

These are just three of more than a hundred forms of arthritis, according to the Arthritis Foundation. More than 40 million Americans, 97 percent over age sixty, have some form of arthritis. Why is it so common? The free radical, wear-and-tear theory of aging (see Chapter 2) may be one answer. Indeed, medical evidence is mounting that free radical wear-and-tear is involved in many forms of arthritis. For instance, in rheumatoid arthritis free radicals strike the synovial membrane, a thin tissue lining the space between the joints of the bones, causing inflammation and pain. In osteoarthritis, free radicals strike proteins in joint cartilage, cutting the protein into fragments that then solidify, decreasing joint mobility.

TREATMENT OF ARTHRITIS BY ANTIOXIDANTS

A free radical scavenging enzyme known as superoxide dimutase (SOD) has been used experimentally, but with good results in humans. In the original pilot study of the substance, nineteen patients suffering from osteoarthritis of the knee joint were injected with 2–3 mg of SOD into the synovial cleft of the knee joint. "After three injections, sixteen of nineteen patients improved."[6] The successful results were duplicated in randomized, double-blind trials conducted separately on groups of patients from Scandinavia, Great Britain, and

Central Europe. The substance "was found to be superior to placebo for clinically relevant parameters like pain, functional improvement in terms of walking ability, and climbing stairs."[7]

The alpha-tocopherol form of vitamin E has also been studied. In one study, 400 IU (one small capsule) of this vitamin was given once a day over a period of six weeks. The patients were able to reduce their intake of painkillers, nonsteroidal anti-inflammatory drugs (NSAIDS).[8] This is important because, at large doses, NSAIDS have a tendency to cause nausea and other stomach upsets.

Belgium and French research collaborators wrote that their data "provide a strong rationale for the therapeutic use of antioxidants . . . most anti-inflammatory drugs have side effects. . . . Antioxidants such as vitamin E are known for their good tolerance, or SOD known for its sustained effect . . . may prolong the pain-free intervals and reduce the need for analgesics."[9]

It stands to reason that if antioxidants are being used successfully in the treatment of various forms of arthritis, they may, if taken before the onset of disease, also delay the onset of many forms of this dread disease by shielding us from free radicals. A leading Brazilian medical researcher, writing in a textbook for doctors titled *Free Radicals and Aging,* goes even further: "The role of free radicals in the intrinsic aging process, as well as in age-related degenerative diseases, seems to be well established. This implies the use of free radical scavengers and antioxidants for prevention and therapy of age-related diseases. Hopefully also, human life span may be prolonged, or at least the periods of illness and suffering during the last years of human life may be shortened."[10]

DIABETES

ETHEL REVERSES DIABETES THROUGH DIET AND EXERCISE

Ethel is a sixty-eight-year-old retired office manager who was referred to me in 1987 because of diabetes. At a routine visit to her gynecologist she was found to have high blood pressure, diabetes, and obesity. During a glucose tolerance test her blood glucose values were 213 mg/100 ml at one hour (normal values are less than 200 mg/100 ml) and 236 mg/100 ml at two hours (normal values are less than 140 mg/100 ml). These abnormally high values indicate that she has diabetes in the early stages. Ethel was quite concerned about these new diagnoses when she came to see me because her mother had suffered from major kidney and circulation problems related to diabetes.

At Ethel's first visit her blood pressure was 180/94, her weight was 185 pounds, and her height was 5 feet, 10 inches. Other than the high blood pressure, her physical examination was normal. However, laboratory tests revealed further problems. The blood triglycerides were 322 mg/100 ml (twice as high as they should be) and the HDL-cholesterol "good guys" were too low.

Because of the diabetes, high blood pressure, and high triglycerides, the dietitian instructed her in our high-carbohydrate, high-fiber diet and I asked her to increase her walking from a minimum amount to two miles per day, six days per week. Ethel enthusiastically endorsed this program. At six weeks she was doing everything we had asked her and we gave her further coaching on diet and exercise.

After three months, Ethel had lost 13 pounds and all her numbers had improved (see Table 6.1). We encouraged her to continue and saw her every two months. By one year she had achieved a nonobese weight (for her, fewer than 165 pounds). Her glucose values were in the normal range, and the HDL cholesterol and triglycerides had improved. We encouraged her to continue the diet and exercise program.

Ethel has come in to see me every three or four months since 1987 and has continued her diet and exercise program. She has maintained a nonobese weight and has not developed diabetes. In 1993 I recommended that she start taking an antioxidant supplement containing beta-carotene, 15,000 IU (9 mg); vitamin C, 1,000 mg; and vitamin E, 800 IU. She continues the high-carbohydrate, high-fiber diet that is rich in vegetables and fruits from the antioxidant honor roll (see Chapter 8).

TABLE 6.1   ETHEL'S SCORECARD

MEASUREMENT	FIRST VISIT	THREE MONTHS	ONE YEAR	GOALS
Weight	185	172	157	150
Blood pressure	180/94	150/88	132/78	<150/90
Glucose*	115	104	86	<110
HDL cholesterol*	30	38	44	≥55
Triglycerides*	322	210	167	<150
Exercise	minimal	12 miles/wk.	12 miles/wk.	12 miles/wk.

* Values are for mg/100 ml.

WHAT YOU NEED TO KNOW ABOUT DIABETES

There are about 14 million people with diabetes in the United States, and their number is increasing daily throughout the world. Only half of those who have diabetes know they have it, according to the American Diabetes Association. The other 7 million diabetics are undiagnosed, but may have dangerous amounts of sugar in their bloodstreams. The danger is this: If you are diabetic your body is unable to break down and use foods properly. That means that excessive amounts of sugar, instead of being burned as energy, accumulate in the blood and spill into the urine. Over time, high levels of sugar cause accelerated aging that can damage the eyes, kidneys, nerves, and arteries and lead to disability and ultimately premature death.[11]

Diabetes develops when the pancreas is unable to produce enough insulin and/or cellular mechanisms called receptor sites aren't working right. Free radical damage to beta cells, the insulin manufacturing sites on the pancreas,[12] and/or free radical damage to insulin receptor sites are two factors that set the stage for diabetes. Think of insulin as a key and the receptor cells as a lock. If the pancreas doesn't make enough insulin, this "key" substance is spread too thin to unlock all the necessary receptor sites. If the receptor sites themselves malfunction, the "locks" cannot open to accept the excess blood sugar into the cells.

Diabetics have twice the rate of heart disease and stroke as non-diabetics. That is why our study, mentioned in Chapter 3, of the protective effects of antioxidants on humans is so important. That study showed that vitamins C and E and beta-carotene delay the oxidation

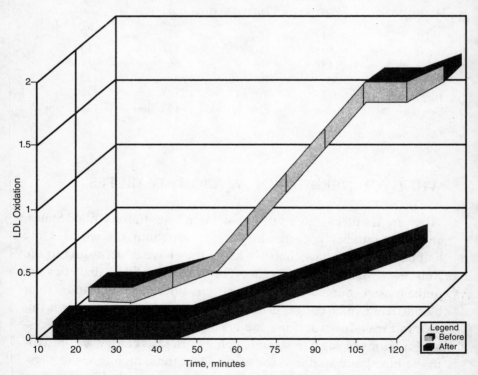

FIGURE 6.1   Rate of oxidation of LDL in diabetics before and after antioxidant treatment. (See Chapter 3.)

of low-density cholesterol that leads to hardening of the arteries. This delay prolongs life and buys diabetics time to get their sugar levels under control. We recommend that diabetics, or anyone at risk of developing diabetes, walk often and do simple upper-body exercises regularly. The reason is that these types of activities increase the receptivity of receptor sites to insulin.

For most people, diabetes is a preventable disease. As my patient Ethel illustrates, most people with a tendency toward diabetes can nip it in the bud with diet and exercise. More than twenty years ago our research group began treating diabetic persons with high-carbohydrate, high-fiber diets. For most people this diet alleviated the need for medication, and many came off of insulin.[13, 14] One of my most successful patients has gone twenty years after stopping insulin treatment and now uses only diet and exercise to manage his diabetes. Thus, intensive diet and exercise reverse diabetes in some adults who develop their diabetes after age forty.

Population studies indicate that high-fiber intake protects from development of diabetes.[13] Low-fat intake also protects from development of diabetes.[13] Thus the regular intake of a diet rich in vegetables and fruits and poor in animal fat is a major defense against the development of diabetes. This diet, of course, would be rich in antioxidants. Human studies also indicate that avoidance of obesity and regular exercise protect against development of diabetes.[15]

PREVENTING COMPLICATIONS AND CONTROLLING DIABETES

A few years ago diabetics received some good news from a landmark medical study. The results of the ten-year, $165 million study called the Diabetes Control and Complications Trial (DCCT) showed that Type I diabetics who kept a tight rein on their blood sugar levels developed fewer and less severe complications than those whose sugar level measurements were under less strict control. Type I diabetics are insulin-dependent. These patients often develop diabetes when they are young. They are usually slim, but not as fit and trim as they should be. They require frequent injections of insulin to lower the high levels of glucose[16] in their bloodstreams. On the other hand, Type II diabetes (sometimes called adult-onset diabetes because that's when the disease appears) is also confusingly known as "non-insulin-dependent diabetes" (NIDDM) because most Type II diabetics control their conditions with diet and exercise alone. However, many Type II diabetics cannot control their blood sugar levels through diet and exercise alone. They either have to take oral medicines to stimulate the release of insulin from the pancreas and to tone up their cells' sensitivity to insulin, or they have to take regular injections of insulin, just like the Type I patients. Since the DCCT study was conducted on Type I patients, one question is, "Do the results pertain to the more numerous Type IIs?" While the two different types of diabetes have different inheritance patterns and other differences, such as age of onset and body weight, both have in common the most important negative about diabetes. The heart of the problem for both groups is that they have too much sugar, in the form of glucose, in their blood. Because of that similarity most experts believe that all diabetics should maintain tight control. As DCCT study chairman Oscar Crofford, M.D., says, "Until a cure is found, intensive diabetes management is the best way to prevent complications."[17]

ANTIOXIDANTS PROTECT AGAINST DEVELOPMENT OF DIABETES

Studies in laboratory animals indicate that use of vitamin E protects from several forms of experimental diabetes. Most forms of experimental diabetes result from free radical damage to the insulin-producing beta cells of the pancreas. Pretreatment of the animals with vitamin E before administering the toxic chemical protects the animals from developing diabetes.[18] Human diabetes of the adult-onset (Type II) type results from a premature aging of the insulin-producing beta cells of the pancreas. The exact mechanisms are unclear. It seems reasonable to speculate that intake of adequate amounts of antioxidants, especially vitamin E, may protect from development of diabetes. This hypothesis is consistent with the available data indicating that the intake of generous amounts of antioxidant-rich plant foods protects against development of diabetes.

ANTIOXIDANT INTAKE PROTECTS AGAINST KIDNEY AND EYE DISEASE IN DIABETES

Oxidation of proteins by free radicals is a major problem in diabetes. High blood sugar levels promote excessive oxidation of proteins in the kidneys, eyes, and other parts of the body.[19] The oxidation of protein sets the stage for damage to the kidneys and the eyes. Recent research indicates that treatment of diabetic individuals with either vitamin C or vitamin E reduces the formation of free radicals and oxidation of protein.[20, 21] Further studies are required but these preliminary studies suggest that regular intake of vitamin C and E will reduce free-radical damage to tissues in diabetes and lessen the likelihood of development of diabetic kidney and eye problems.[21]

MAURY'S DIARY

In 1994 I was diagnosed as having adult-onset, Type II diabetes. At first I was able to control the disease with pills to stimulate my pancreas to produce more insulin. Unfortunately, the disease progressed rather rapidly to the point that I had to take insulin shots twice a day. That's when I started learning about what foods to eat, the value of exercise, and the importance of monitoring my blood sugar levels.

I now check my blood sugar several times a day with one of the nifty new monitoring devices that require only a droplet of blood. These monitors report on the sugar content of the blood in less than a minute. To get the recommended "hanging droplet" for the test, I use a spring-propelled autolancet to prick one of my fingers. I do this at least twice a day, often more. At first I noticed that my blood droplets didn't flow quickly. In fact, they moved like sludge.

Motivated, I began taking Dr. Anderson's recommended antioxidant supplements and improved my diet to include at least five servings of fruit and/or vegetables a day. The results were quick and dramatic. When I lance my finger now the blood squirts out—no more artery-clogging sludge. Best of all, my insulin requirements have been reduced by a third. I feel more alive and energetic. My ability to concentrate has improved. I believe that Dr. Anderson's Antioxidant, Antiaging Health Program is protecting me from the complications of diabetes and from an early death.

REDUCE BLOOD SUGAR

Besides exercise, the most important factors in controlling blood sugar levels are what and how often you eat. The antioxidant-phytochemical-rich diet detailed in Chapter 8 is high in fiber and low in fat. Fiber, which is found in fruits, vegetables, nuts, and whole grains, slows digestion of carbohydrates, thus preventing sudden jumps of glucose in the blood. Fat, which contains more calories gram for gram than carbohydrate or protein, should be cut to 30 percent of everyone's dietary intake, but diabetics or those at risk for diabetes should make even more stringent cuts. People at risk for diabetes should cut their fat intake to 25 percent or less of total calories, and those with diabetes, especially the overweight, should cut fat intake to 20 percent or less. Following these suggestions should help anyone lose excess weight, an especially important goal for diabetics or those at risk of diabetes.

I, (Dr. Anderson) know that high-fiber diets lower blood sugar because of many studies accomplished by the Metabolic Research Group at the Veterans Affairs Medical Center and University of Kentucky at Lexington. Details of one of our recent high-fiber studies appeared in the July 1995 issue of the research journal *Metabolism*.[22] We explained how we tested the effects of high- and low-fiber meals on the after-meal levels of serum glucose, insulin, fats, and proteins in ten nonobese, middle-aged men. The volunteers ate weight-maintaining diets of commonly available foods. By design, their total fiber intakes in the high-fiber diet were about eightfold higher than in the low-fiber one. One way we achieved the increase in fiber was including psyllium (the regular orange-flavored Metamucil brand, manufactured by Procter & Gamble), which is marketed as a laxative. In the high-fiber diet the men drank 3.4 gm of psyllium with every meal. Subjects tolerated the dose quite well. This study, and others like it,[23] confirmed the important effect of dietary fiber on after-meal blood glucose and insulin responses. That's one reason I recommend that people on my antioxidant, antiaging program intake at least 20 to 35 gm of fiber a day. This amount can be eaten by just having three servings of vegetables per day and two of fruit. If you consistently miss achieving this level of fruit and vegetable intake, consider taking psyllium as the study volunteers did.

Other goals for helping diabetics on my antiaging food plan include helping them:

- maintain as near normal blood glucose and blood pressure levels as possible;
- achieve the best possible blood serum cholesterol and triglycerides levels;
- provide adequate calories to allow the maintenance of a healthy, active life.[24]

EYE DISEASES

WHAT YOU NEED TO KNOW ABOUT YOUR EYES

As we get older, all of us become more susceptible to vision problems. Scientists have discovered that free radicals play important preventive roles in two of the most prevalent causes of vision impairment in older adults—cataracts and a condition called age-related macular degeneration (ARMD).[25]

CATARACTS

This sight-stealing disease is the leading cause of blindness and visual impairment in the world. Some 46 percent of all individuals aged seventy-five to eighty-five have cataracts.[26] As a result, cataract surgery has become the most common surgical procedure among people who are sixty-five years of age or older.[27] Cataracts occur when opaque areas develop within the normally transparent lens of the eye. "Basic research studies have shown that oxidative mechanisms probably play an important role in cataract development, perhaps by damaging the lens," writes Dr. William Christian, Jr., of Harvard Medical School.[28]

"While the only treatment for cataract may indeed be surgery, it is not the only 'remedy.' A patient wishing to prevent cataracts must be willing to make dietary changes and use antioxidant supplements before the cataract appears," states Dr. James Heffley, editor of the *Journal of Applied Nutrition* and director of nutrition at the Nutrition Counseling Service, Austin, Texas.

"Our research shows there is a lower risk of developing cataracts in people who consume a lot of vitamin C in their diet," confimed Dr. Allen Taylor, Director of the Lens Nutrition and Ageing Division of the U.S. Department of Agriculture's Research Center on Aging (at Tufts University, Boston). Added Linda Davis Kyle, an internationally published health writer who has served on the board of directors of the Prevent Blindness foundation since 1989, "Research has revealed that vitamin E is a team player. Vitamin E, vitamin C, and carotenoids create a protective micro-environment in the lens tissue that delays the development of cataracts."[29]

The condition occurring when the lens loses some of its clarity is called a cataract. Cataracts are age-related. Most occur in people who are in their sixties or seventies, though some unlucky people have developed cataracts as early as their forties. During the early stages of a cataract, the problem is treated with eyeglass lens adjustments and the use of sunglasses. Years can pass before the cataract becomes so mature that surgery is necessary. "Cataract surgery has evolved into one of the most successful operations ever performed," says eye expert James Collins, a practicing ophthalmologist who is medical director of the Center for Eye Care on Long Island, New York. "There is usually better than a 95 percent chance of vision being restored to precataract conditions."[30]

AGE-RELATED MACULAR DEGENERATION

Age-related macular degeneration (ARMD) is a degenerative process that is the leading cause of blindness for people over sixty years of age. "If left untreated, 7.5 million American adults will suffer vision loss from ARMD by the year 2020,"[31] states Dr. Stuart P. Richer, coinvestigator in the U.S. Veterans Administration Pacific University Multicenter ARMD Study. This destructive eye disease occurs in a highly specialized part of the retina called the macula lutea, a yellowish region on the retina responsible for providing the detailed central vision needed for such tasks as reading, sewing, television viewing, or woodworking.

There are two types of ARMD: "dry," which accounts for 80 percent of all cases, and "wet," which accounts for the rest. The "wet" variety is the more serious of the two. Dry ARMD can be treated with laser surgery if diagnosed and treated early, but there is no proven form of treatment for wet ARMD.[32] Wet ARMD accounts for 90 percent of all severe visual loss attributed to ARMD. Reduction of vision is rapid. Because of the seriousness and lack of treatment methods for wet ARMD, vision experts are increasingly recommending antioxidant therapy as a means of prevention.

PREVENTION OF CATARACTS AND ARMD

Mom was right! Eat your vegetables. Nutritional studies offer evidence that individuals with a high intake of fruit and vegetables rich in vitamin A have a 40 percent reduction of risk for ARMD.[33] Studies also indicate that cataract patients tend to have low antioxidant levels in their bloodstreams[34] and that taking higher levels of antioxidants, especially higher levels of vitamin C, may postpone the onset of cataracts. "Results show that subjects with high levels of at least two of the three vitamins (vitamin E, vitamin C, or carotenoids) are at reduced risk of cataract," wrote Dr. Paul F. Jacques and his colleagues at the USDA's Human Nutrition Research Center on Aging at Tufts University, in an article published in *The Archives of Ophthalmology*.[35] Writing in *The Journal of the American Medical Association* about a study conducted by five ophthalmology centers throughout the United States, Dr. Johanna M. Seddon of the Massachusetts Eye and Ear Infirmary and the Harvard University School of Health and several of her colleagues specifically mentioned the beneficial effects of two specific vegetables: "A higher frequency of intake of spinach or collard greens was associated with a substantially lower risk for ARMD."[36]

TAKE YOUR SUPPLEMENTS

The large-scale cancer study in Linxian, China, also included a smaller study of the impact of antioxidants on cataracts. One result was that people aged sixty-five to seventy-four who took multivitamin supplements that included beta-carotene, vitamin C, and vitamin E "at doses 1½ to 3 times the [U.S.] recommended daily allowance"[37] were found to have a 35 percent reduced risk of cataracts. Another study, this one of 17,774 U.S. physicians, concluded that those "who took multivitamin supplements [containing antioxidant vitamins and minerals] tended to experience a decreased risk of cataract."[38]

Supplements are necessary because most people aren't able to follow an ideal diet day after day. A recent study of healthy people over age fifty-five who ate a diet considered normal for adults found that three of four of the participants were deficient in two or more of the antioxidants (such as vitamin C and beta-carotene) thought to be important to eye health. Almost all participants in the study fell short on at least one of the antioxidants, according to study leader Michael S. Kaminski. Dr. Kaminski was one of four authors (the others were Drs. Anita M. Van Der Hagen, Diane P. Yolton, and Robert

L. Yolton) who collaborated in an article in the *Journal of the American Optometric Association* saying that "it is possible that the damage [from ARMD] could be prevented or moderated by supplementing the diet with specific antioxidant vitamins and minerals that enhance the body's natural defenses against free radicals. . . . It seems reasonable to suggest supplementation to most or all patients. . . ."[39]

TO SUM UP

- Simple dietary changes found in Chapter 8 can help you avoid or at least delay the arrival of degenerative conditions such as aging skin, arthritis, diabetes, and vision problems.
- Free radicals attack our skin, the body's largest organ, causing "crow's-feet" and wrinkles.
- Antioxidants, especially vitamin E, protect the protein in our skin.
- Although cosmetics companies add vitamin E and other antioxidants to lotions, moisturizing agents, and other beauty products, except for vitamin E in suntanning lotions, there is little research to confirm that the manufacturers add enough antioxidants to make a difference.
- There are more than a hundred forms of arthritis. Antioxidants have been used with good results experimentally in humans, especially in those with osteoarthritis of the knee.
- Antioxidants combat free radical attacks that can cause inflammation and pain, and antioxidants may prevent or delay the occurrence of arthritis in its many forms.
- Seven million Americans are in great danger healthwise because they are undiagnosed diabetics.
- The DCCT, a landmark research study, confirms that diabetics need to control the amount of sugar in their blood to prevent complications such as damage to their eyes, heart, kidneys, nerves, and arteries in their later years.
- Medical research has shown that vitamins C and E and beta-

carotene protect low-density cholesterol from oxidation. Adequate amounts of these nutrients delay the process known as hardening of the arteries and thus can extend the life span of many individuals.

- Diabetics and others at risk for heart problems, should eat high-fiber diets such as those explained in the antioxidant, antiaging food program in Chapter 8.
- We become more susceptible to vision problems as we grow older.
- The most common visual problem, cataracts, can be treated surgically with a 95 percent success rate.
- Since cataracts patients usually have low antioxidant levels, they should make a concentrated effort to include more fruits and vegetables in their diets and should take multivitamin antioxidant supplements.

WHAT YOU CAN DO RIGHT NOW

- Eat at least two servings of fruit and three of vegetables every day.
- Take antioxidant supplements. You'll find advice on what antioxidants to take and in what amounts in Chapter 8.
- If you are age fifty or older or if you have diabetes, have your eyes checked by an ophthalmologist or optometrist at least once a year.
- Walk often and do simple upper-body exercises regularly.
- Wear appropriate protective eyewear such as wraparound goggles when using tools or playing sports such as racquetball that may put your eyes in danger.
- Be sure to carefully read all labels, note expiration dates, and understand the directions for use on any substance you plan to put into your eyes. Many eye injuries occur when people mistakenly use various chemicals and medications as eyewashes or home treatments.

The Joys of Soy: Reduced Risks for Heart Disease, Cancer, and Osteoporosis

MARCIE PROTECTS HERSELF FROM BREAST CANCER, HEART DISEASE, AND OSTEOPOROSIS

Marcie is a fifty-eight-year-old highly successful real estate agent who came to see me because of high blood cholesterol levels. Her recent blood cholesterol values had been 283 mg/100 ml. Two years previously she had surgery for breast cancer and subsequently received chemotherapy. Although she had an excellent prognosis from her breast cancer, she could not take estrogen replacement. She was concerned about her high blood cholesterol levels and the risk of developing osteoporosis. Her mother and one aunt had moderately severe osteoporosis, and she wanted to do everything she could to prevent this problem.

The history and the physical examination for Marcie indicated that she was in good general health. She had no evidence of heart disease, recurrent breast cancer, or osteoporosis. Except for her blood cholesterol and LDL cholesterol values (see initial values in Table 7.1), the laboratory studies revealed no abnormalities.

Marcie's program was tailored to her needs as follows:*

- *antioxidant food plan:* at least two servings of soy protein (20 gm) per day and at least five servings of antioxidant-rich vegetables and fruits;
- *exercise plan:* walking two miles daily for six days per week and doing upper-body exercises several days weekly;
- *antioxidant supplementation:* two capsules twice daily;
- *multiple vitamin-mineral supplementation:* one capsule without iron daily.

Because there was no family or personal history of premature vascular disease, I did not recommend that she take additional folic acid, vitamin B_6, and vitamin B_{12}. However, to reduce risk for osteoporosis, I recommended taking 1,500 mg of elemental calcium daily. Because of her high blood cholesterol value, I also recommended that she take psyllium powder (which lowers blood cholesterol) and wrote a prescription for bile acid binding tablets (two tablets twice daily).

Marcie liked the new food plan and followed it carefully; she found new and innovative ways to work soy protein into the menu for her husband and herself. She increased her level of exercise to walking two miles daily and started using a cross-training machine. She took her supplements, psyllium powder, and bile acid binding tablets regularly. After three months her blood lipids showed an excellent response and were close to the desirable values for her. She continues to follow this program closely.

TABLE 7.1   MARCIE'S SCORECARD

MEASUREMENT	INITIAL	THREE MONTHS	GOALS
Blood cholesterol	274	216	≤200
LDL cholesterol	189	136	≤130
HDL cholesterol	65	57	≥55
Triglycerides	98	115	≤150

* See Table 8.1 for more details.

IMPORTANCE OF SOY THROUGHOUT THE WORLD

Asian diets, such as those in Japan and China, are usually lower in total and saturated fat and are higher in dietary fiber than most Western diets. These dietary differences have been used to explain the lower rates of coronary heart disease, breast cancer, prostate cancer, colon cancer, and osteoporosis in Asian people compared to Western people.[1] Recent research, however, suggests that differences in the intake of soybean products also may contribute to the much lower rates of "Western diseases" among Asian people.

Whenever epidemiologic, between-population comparisons are made, the intake of animal protein is strongly associated with Western diseases, while the intake of vegetable, or soybean, protein is correlated inversely. In other words, the intake of large amounts of animal protein appears to provide a foundation for Western diseases, while the intake of soy protein appears to provide protection.[1]

Soybeans are important sources of certain phytochemicals or plant chemicals. New and exciting research demonstrates that many phytochemicals have potent anticancer and antioxidant properties. Other phytochemicals, such as the tocotrienols, various building blocks of vitamin E, have important cholesterol-lowering effects. Soybeans are rich sources of a type of phytochemical classified as isoflavones, which have important preventive actions with respect to coronary heart disease, breast cancer, prostate cancer, and osteoporosis.[1-3] We will review some of this fast-breaking information.

SOY ISOFLAVONES

For thousands of years witch doctors, medicine men, midwives, shamans, herbalists, and knowledgeable people have used certain plants, herbs, or spices for protective, enabling, or curative effects. Digitalis, which comes from the foxglove plant and is used to treat congestive heart failure, is one example. There are tens of thousands of phytochemicals, and most have not yet been clearly identified. Soybeans are rich sources of many different phytochemicals. Isoflavones, a type of phytochemical, may be unique to soybeans, since they have not been clearly identified in other types of plant foods.

In the past ten years isoflavones have attracted major attention because of their important chemical properties. First, and relevant to this book, soy isoflavones are potent antioxidants that are carried by lipid particles in the bloodstream and act to prevent oxidation of lipid particles and their contribution to hardening of the arteries (see Chapter 3). Second, soy isoflavones appear to be the major component of soy protein, which lowers blood cholesterol levels.[2] Third, studies using several types of experimental animals indicate that soy isoflavones protect against developing breast cancer.[4] Fourth, soy isoflavones prevent the growth of human breast cancer cells in the test tube.[3] Fifth, these soy compounds prevent formation of new blood vessels, technically called angiogenesis, in experimental animals and in test tubes.[3] Inhibition of new blood vessel formation would slow growth of tumors in the body, since rapidly growing cells need new blood vessels. Sixth, soy isoflavones inhibit development of prostate cancer in animals.[3] Seventh, animal experiments indicate that soy compounds protect against osteoporosis.[5]

There are two major isoflavones in soy products, genistein and daidzein. When scientists determined the chemical structure of these soy phytochemicals they found that they resembled estradiole (the major human female estrogen) and tamoxifen (an antiestrogen used to prevent the spread of human breast cancer). Genistein has a curious mix of antiestrogen and proestrogen effects. Genistein protects against development of breast cancer in animal models and perhaps in humans. Genistein acts like estrogen in women who are postmenopausal, thus decreasing menopausal symptoms. It also may protect from development of osteoporosis. Mother Nature was very clever in developing this phytochemical, which appears to do all the right things for women.[6] In addition to these benefits, soy isoflavones lower blood cholesterol levels in women and men and, as a bonus for men, may protect from prostate and colon cancer.[3]

Soy protein provides about 2 mg of isoflavones per gram of protein. Many Asian people obtain 80 to 120 mg per day of these important soy compounds from their diet, while many Western people have negligible intakes of them. In fact, one study in Great Britain indicated that average intake there was fewer than 1 mg per day.[3] Not enough information is available to recommend a desirable level of intake. Our research on effects of soy protein on blood cholesterol levels suggest that at least 30 to 50 mg per day may be required; this would be the amount of isoflavones contained in 15 to 25 g (0.5 to 1 oz.) of soy protein per day.

While the importance of soy isoflavones is still under investigation, a daily intake of soy protein products rich in these isoflavones is desirable. Most soy products, except those containing soy protein concentrate, are excellent sources of isoflavones. Unfortunately, the soy protein concentrate currently used to make burgers and other meat substitutes has only small amounts of soy isoflavones. In contrast, soy milk or soy beverage, soy flour, tofu, textured soy protein, and isolated soy protein are rich in isoflavones and provide about 2 mg of isoflavones per gram of protein. Our research group is performing clinical trials to examine the cholesterol-lowering effects of currently available soy protein products. Until further information is available, we recommend choosing soy protein products rich in isoflavones, such as soy milk (beverage), soy flour, tofu, textured soy protein, and isolated soy protein.

RISK FOR HEART DISEASE

High intakes of animal protein are associated with high rates of coronary heart disease. While conventional wisdom attributes this association to the saturated fat content of animal protein, unconventional thinking wonders whether the animal protein itself may contribute to hardening of the arteries. On the flip side, low intakes of animal protein with generous intakes of soy protein are associated with low rates of coronary heart disease. Emerging evidence suggests that soy protein, with its isoflavone content, may be the protector in these soybean-rich diets. Soy protein intake significantly decreases blood cholesterol levels, and soy isoflavones have important antioxidant properties.

SOY PROTEIN AND BLOOD LIPID LEVELS

The effects of soy protein intake on serum cholesterol levels have been controversial.[7] Because my own preliminary analysis of the studies suggested that soy protein intake had a definite effect on serum cholesterol levels, my associates and I carefully reviewed and analyzed previous human studies. This detailed statistical analysis is called a meta-analysis. First, we assembled all the studies published in the world literature. Next, we determined what information should be analyzed from these studies. Third, we tabulated all the data. Next, we entered all the data into a special computer program and performed a number of complicated statistical analyses. Finally, we summarized the results into a scientific paper published in *The New England Journal of Medicine (NEJ).*[2]

We analyzed 38 studies, which included 730 research volunteers. Some studies included only 5 people; the average study included 19 volunteers. While 34 studies reported that soy protein intake decreased cholesterol in the blood, most of the decreases did not reach the level of statistical significance accepted by scientists. However, the meta-analysis allowed us to combine results as though all 730 people had participated in one big study. Instead of analyzing results for 19 volunteers, we could analyze results for 730 people. This enabled us to draw stronger conclusions than previously possible.

Our meta-analysis indicates that soy protein intake decreases serum cholesterol levels by 9.3 percent. Serum LDL cholesterol levels decreased 12.9 percent and serum triglycerides decreased 10.5 percent. All of these changes were considered to be highly significant by medical researchers. As a bonus, soy protein tends to increase serum HDL cholesterol levels by 2.4 percent, although this increase was not statistically significant. Thus the daily intake of soy protein changes all the serum lipid levels in a favorable direction. Of course, as pointed out in Chapter 3, elevated values for serum cholesterol, LDL cholesterol, and triglycerides increase risk for hardening of the arteries while, as you know, high serum levels of HDL cholesterol decrease risk for coronary heart disease.

In our analysis, the average intake of soy protein was 47 g per day. The bad news is that this is the amount of soy protein in one pound of tofu or six glasses of soy beverage (soy milk) or four tablespoons of isolated soy protein. Many of us would find it difficult to eat this much tofu or drink this much soy milk. The good news is that 40 percent of the studies used 31 g of soy protein or less. We estimate that 20 g of soy protein or two servings will provide enough soy protein and isoflavones to significantly decrease serum cholesterol levels. In the medical community there is a consensus that every 1 percent reduction in serum cholesterol level decreases risk for coronary heart disease by 2 to 3 percent.[8] If 20 g of soy protein decreased serum cholesterol levels by 6 to 8 percent, this would reduce risk of coronary heart disease by 12 to 24 percent. Soy protein would further decrease risk through the decrease in serum triglycerides and the increase in serum HDL cholesterol levels.

Our meta-analysis firmly establishes the benefits of soy protein for lowering serum cholesterol levels. Two major questions remain: How much soy protein is necessary to reduce the serum cholesterol levels? What are the mechanisms by which soy protein decreases serum cholesterol levels? We are conducting further research to answer these and other questions.

MONKEY BUSINESS

Some of the most illuminating studies on soy protein and risk of coronary heart disease have been conducted with monkeys. Dr. Tom Clarkson and associates at Bowman Gray School of Medicine in Winston-Salem, North Carolina, have examined not only the effects of soy protein with and without isoflavones but also the effects of soy protein intake on the function of blood vessels. Figure 7.1 summarizes the results of their studies comparing soy protein rich in isoflavones (+ isoflavones) and soy protein from which the

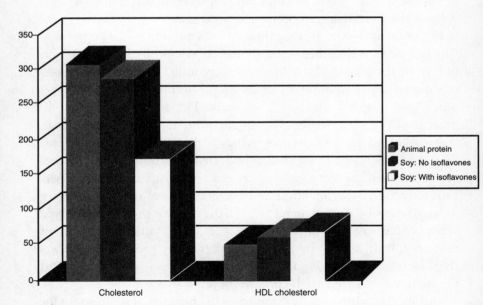

FIGURE 7.1   Comparison of the Effects of Animal Protein, Soy Protein with Isoflavones, and Soy Protein with No Isoflavones on Serum Cholesterol and HDL Cholesterol Levels in Monkeys[9]

isoflavones had been extracted (– isoflavones). Most of the choles-terol-lowering effects are associated with the isoflavone content, since soy protein-rich isoflavones decreased serum cholesterol levels by 35 percent while soy protein without isoflavones decreased serum cholesterol levels by only 5 percent. However, both soy pro-teins were accompanied by an increase in HDL cholesterol levels.[9] Further studies are required to sort out these differing effects.

In addition to the favorable effects of isoflavone-rich soy proteins on serum lipids, these proteins also protect LDL from oxidation and improve the function of blood vessels. Recent studies from Dr. Clarkson and associates demonstrate that feeding isoflavone-rich soy proteins to monkeys preserves the ability of blood vessels to di-late properly in response to the need for more blood supply. Thus soy proteins rich in isoflavones have a number of favorable effects in monkeys and probably offer similar benefits to humans.

BREAST CANCER RISK

Breast cancer is the second most common cancer in Western women but has a much lower incidence among women in Third World and Asian countries. These differences appear related to environmental, rather than genetic factors, since Asian women who migrate to Western countries develop breast cancer at rates similar to Western women within one generation. Among other differences between Western countries and Asian countries such as Japan and China, the intake of soy protein is much higher in these Asian countries than in Western countries. Several epidemiologic studies, or population comparison studies, suggest that the intake of soy protein is related to a reduced risk for developing breast cancer.[1] The isoflavones ap-pear to be the active ingredients of soy protein products that lower this breast cancer risk.

In studies of breast cancer in animals, intake of soy protein or of soy isoflavones appears to protect against development of breast cancer. These studies are not conclusive, however, since protection was reported in only five of eight studies.[1] More recent studies suggest that the major soy isoflavone genistein protects against development of breast cancer in animals. Recent studies suggest that genistein inhibits the growth of human breast cancer cells, at least in test tubes.[4]

PROSTATE AND OTHER CANCERS

The soy isoflavone genistein is a potent antioxidant and also inhibits a number of chemical reactions in the body. Genistein slows activity of several proteins that speed up tumor growth, and decreases new blood vessel formation, which would limit the ability of tumors to grow rapidly. This slowing process tends to protect against the growth of certain cancers, especially those related to hormone levels such as breast and prostate cancer.[3]

Epidemiologic studies suggest that Oriental men who consume generous amounts of soy protein have lower rates of prostate cancer than Western men who consume negligible amounts of soy protein. Several studies in experimental animals suggest that soy protein protects from development of prostate cancer in animal models. In addition, genistein inhibits the growth of prostate cancer cells in the test tube.[3]

The potential protective effects of soy protein and soy isoflavones are intriguing and require much further study. The potential benefits for women who cannot or do not wish to take estrogen replacement or for women with strong family histories of breast cancer seem fairly large. Certainly any risks from increasing soy protein intake appear to be less that that of taking the antiestrogen tamoxifen, which is being used in chemoprevention trials for breast cancer.

OSTEOPOROSIS

Asian women have less osteoporosis than Western women even though the calcium intake of Asian women is lower. Some researchers suggest that the intake of soy protein with its isoflavones contributes to this protection from osteoporosis.[1] The soy isoflavones have weak proestrogen effects, which might contribute to this favorable effect on bone. Of interest, use of the antiestrogen tamoxifen decreases rates of osteoporosis. Recent animal studies indicate that soy protein intake or soy isoflavone feeding slows the progression of osteoporosis in a rat model for osteoporosis.[5] Further studies are required to examine the relationship between soy protein and isoflavones and osteoporosis.

OTHER DISEASES

The proestrogen and antiestrogen effects of the soy isoflavones are puzzling and still under examination. For comparative purposes, the various effects of soy protein, estrogens, and tamoxifen on serum lipids are summarized in Table 7.2. Human estrogens such as estradiole decrease serum cholesterol and LDL cholesterol. Tamoxifen and soy protein have similar effects. However, estradiole and tamoxifen increase serum triglyceride values, while soy protein lowers these values. All three of these decrease the risk of heart attack and osteoporosis. However, use of human estrogens increases the risk of developing breast cancer, while use of tamoxifen and, presumably, use of soy protein decreases the risk of breast cancer. Because of the similarities between the action of soy protein and the estradiole and tamoxifen compounds, we postulate that the soy isoflavones may be responsible for most of these effects. Studies in the laboratory and with monkeys support the suggestion that much of the effects of soy proteins may be related to their isoflavone content.[3, 4]

TABLE 7.2   HEALTH BENEFITS OF SOY PROTEIN COMPARED TO ESTRADIOLE AND TAMOXIFEN

PARAMETER	ESTRADIOLE	TAMOXIFEN	SOY PROTEIN
Serum cholesterol	Decreases	Decreases	Decreases
Serum LDL cholesterol	Decreases	Decreases	Decreases
Serum HDL cholesterol	Unchanged	Unchanged	Unchanged
Serum triglycerides	Increases	Increases	Decreases
Risk of heart attack	Decreases	Decreases	Decreases
Risk for breast cancer	Increases	Decreases	Decreases
Risk of osteoporosis	Decreases	Decreases	Decreases

Recent 'suggest that regular intake of soy protein with its isoflavones may reduce the symptoms or problems related to estrogen deficiency in women who have had their ovaries removed or are postmenopausal.[6] Further research is being conducted in this important area. Finally, and relevant to this book, recent research in animals suggests that substituting soy protein for animal protein can increase the life span by 13 percent. Thus soy protein and its isoflavones have many health-promoting activities.

JIM'S DIARY

Since the early days I have been a guinea pig and performed all our oat bran, bean, psyllium, and other experiments on myself first. Also, I try to practice what I preach. In July 1995, when I learned that *The New England Journal of Medicine* was going to publish our article, I got serious about the use of soy protein. I purchased tofu, soy beverage (soy milk), soy flour, and textured soy protein. I obtained frozen soyburgers and started using taco mix, sloppy joe mix, and other easy-to-prepare soy protein products. The most popular items I have encountered are the soy muffins. I have made banana nut soy muffins, apple soy muffins, and blueberry soy muffins; my recipes are in Chapter 9. These include soy flour and soy beverage and are popular even with picky eaters. Also I have grown to love vegetable tofu stir-fry. Okay, Jim, how much soy protein do you really eat? Honestly, I eat two servings per day. This includes two muffins at lunch and one "power" bar containing 9 g of soy protein at about three or four o'clock in the afternoon. While I am in the low-risk category according to the listing at the end of this chapter, I am eating soy protein at the high level. And I am truly enjoying it.

PRACTICAL IMPLICATIONS

To get the full benefits of your antioxidant, antiaging program you should begin identifying ways to incorporate soy protein into your diet. One way to do this is to use soy beverage (soy milk) in your cooking and baking. Start incorporating soy flour into your pancakes, waffles, quick breads, and casseroles. Soy beverage and soy flour make great muffins (see the recipes in Chapter 9). As you develop the taste, try using tofu in a stir-fry. Slip small cubes of extra-firm tofu in with cubes of chicken, and your family and friends won't even notice it. Or, for extra insurance, eat a nutrition bar with soy protein. I have a Benefit bar (Health Management Resources, Boston) every day and get in 9 g of soy protein in a very enjoyable way.

Dr. Anderson's Antioxidant, Antiaging Health Program recommends that you include at least one serving of soy protein per day; this should provide about 8 to 10 g of soy protein and about 16 to 20 mgs of isoflavones per day. Chapter 9 outlines specific suggestions for getting in this amount of soy protein. Certain persons should try to get in at least 20 g of soy protein or 40 mg of isoflavones per day. These individuals are postmenopausal women who do not take estrogens, women with a personal history of breast cancer, and women with a strong family history of breast cancer. Men and women with coronary heart disease should also consume at least 20 g of soy protein with 40 mg of isoflavones per day.

Is it okay to use isoflavone supplements, to take a capsule with 20 mg of genistein or 20 mg of isoflavones? In my assessment, the jury is still out on this subject, and *I do not recommend it.* My reasoning is as follows: The soybean is a storehouse of health-promoting phytochemicals, including the isoflavones. While many of the benefits appear related to genistein or other isoflavones, we do not know whether these are the major health-promoting compounds in soybeans. Most of the health benefits that have been recognized in Asian populations are related to intake of the whole soybean or the soybean "cheese" or tofu, which provides most of the soybean constituents except the oil. Since isoflavones were discovered fifty years ago and genistein was identified twenty years ago, they have not been added to food products or tested in humans. Until we have further information, I recommend obtaining your isoflavones from the soy protein products available, which maintain the whole array of phytochemicals in the balanced way that Mother Nature packaged them.

TO SUM UP

- Populations who use generous amounts of soy protein in their diet have lower rates of heart attack, breast cancer, prostate cancer, colon cancer, and osteoporosis than Western people who have low intakes of soy protein.
- Regular intake of soy protein significantly decreases serum levels of cholesterol, LDL ("bad guy") cholesterol, and triglycerides while slightly increasing serum HDL ("good guy") cholesterol levels.
- Soy protein products are rich in phytochemicals called isoflavones. These compounds have important effects on a number of processes in the body.
- Animal experiments show that feeding soy protein or soy isoflavones decreases development of breast cancer. In the test tube, soy isoflavones decrease growth of human breast cancer cells.
- Asian women have less osteoporosis than Western women despite a lower calcium intake. Some research suggests that soy protein

and soy isoflavones in the diet protect from osteoporosis in humans. Animal studies indicate that feeding soy protein or administering soy isoflavones decreases development of osteoporosis.

WHAT YOU CAN DO

GENERAL PREVENTION

If you are in good general health and do not have any of the risks for heart attack outlined in Chapter 3 and do not have a family history of breast cancer:

• Obtain seven servings of soy protein per week. This will give you an average of 8 g of soy protein and 16 g of soy isoflavones per day. You can obtain this amount from 8 oz. of soy beverage per day, two soy muffins per day (as I do), two servings of tofu four times weekly, four soyburgers per week, or 1 tablespoon (14 g) of isolated soy protein stirred into a beverage daily.

TAILORED PROTECTION

If you have risk factors for heart disease (see Chapter 3) or have a family history of breast cancer (in a mother, aunt, or sister):

• Obtain fourteen servings of soy protein per week. This will give you an average of 16 g of soy protein and 32 g of soy isoflavones per day. You will need to develop a routine, as I have, of using soy products regularly. This could include the daily intake of two soy muffins (8 to 10 g), use of a soy nutrition bar (9 g), or use of a soy beverage (8 g). Incorporate tofu and soyburgers into this program.

DISEASE REVERSAL

If you have a history of breast cancer you should use three servings of soy protein per day to get in 24 g of soy protein and 48 g of soy isoflavones per day. If you have heart disease you should use two to three servings of soy protein per day.

• The most practical way to achieve this level of soy protein is to incorporate isolated soy protein powder into a beverage. Two scoops or two heaping tablespoons provide 20 g per day. Then you can get the additional amount from other soy products as outlined above.

JIM'S DIARY

About ten years ago I had dinner with vegetarian friends in Toronto. We went to a Chinese restaurant that served more than twelve different types of bean curd. My friends were in "hog heaven" because of the wide variety of tofu-type products offered. I must admit that I was less enthusiastic but was a good sport. As I tried these various types of bean products, I found that I was enjoying them. Since then I have incorporated more tofu into my diet and have developed a real taste for tofu prepared in a variety of different ways. This interest and admiration for tofu have served me well in the past year, since our research has led to use of soy protein to lower cholesterol and reduce kidney disease in diabetes. In October 1995 I was invited to present our research on soy protein and blood lipids at an international nutrition conference in Beijing, China. After the meeting I was able to visit two other cities in China. During these two weeks in China I had tofu at least twice a day. I really enjoyed the different dishes and flavors. Now stir-fried tofu, tofu in spaghetti sauce, and tofu in other ways are some of my favorite foods. As a result, I have developed a number of tofu and soy protein recipes for you to try.

8

Your Antioxidant Food and Supplement Program

JIM'S PERSONAL HEALTH REGIMEN

Since starting my oat bran research in 1977, I have followed a diet and exercise program to lower my blood cholesterol and reduce my risk of heart attack and stroke. My father developed hypertension in his thirties and had a stroke at age thirty-eight; all of his male relatives had died of strokes in their fifties and early sixties. For almost twenty years I have eaten a high-carbohydrate, high-fiber (HCF) diet. In 1977 I added oat bran and still have oatmeal daily. For eighteen years I have had two oat bran muffins for lunch five days weekly. I still use oat bran cereal as my favorite cold cereal. Since 1985 I have eaten at least five servings of vegetables and fruits daily, and I average forty-five to fifty servings per week. I also began taking one enteric-coated aspirin daily. Since 1985 I have walked an average of twenty-five miles per week.

In 1990 our research led us to antioxidants. Research in diabetes indicated that persons with diabetes were more susceptible to free radical damage (oxidation) of blood fat particles, which set the stage for early and rapidly developing hardening of the arteries. In 1990 I started taking antioxidant supplements daily. As the research on antioxidants emerged, I started using more antioxidants and recommending them for my patients. About three years ago I started eating one-half ounce of nuts at least four times weekly, and about two years ago I started having meals cooked with at least one-fourth tea-spoon of minced garlic at least four times a week.

As our soy research developed, in 1994 I began adding soy protein to my diet. Daily, I have at least two servings of soy products (18 g of soy protein), and several days per week I have an additional 15 to 20 g. Now my favorite evening meal is vegetable stir-fry with tofu; second would be spaghetti with mushroom-tofu sauce.

In the fall of 1995 I started using 1.5 to 3 mg melatonin and Pyc-nogenol daily. I don't routinely recommend them but think they are relatively safe. (See Table 8.1 for recommendations for people with special needs.) During my two-week trip to China I purchased green tea and now have at least two cups daily.

As you examine Table 8.1 you'll see that I'm following the tailored protection program. My dietary fiber intake is about 35 g per day and includes two servings of psyllium to keep my blood cholesterol values below 200 mg/dl. I have about seven servings of vegetables and fruits daily. My fat intake is about 25 percent of calories; I still indulge in one doughnut per week, one or two desserts, and some miscellaneous fat that falls into my path. I only eat fish about twice monthly but take two fish oil capsules daily. I average the following intakes: two to two and a half servings of soy protein daily, four serv-ings of garlic weekly, three cups of green tea daily, four handfuls of nuts weekly, twelve to twenty large purple grapes or four ounces of grape juice daily, and twelve ounces of vegetable juice daily.

For exercise, my program includes twenty miles of walking weekly and forty minutes on the E-force exercise machine per week.

My supplements include one multivitamin and mineral capsule without iron daily; two antioxidant capsules twice daily to provide a total of 20,000 IU (12 mg) beta-carotene, 1,000 mg vitamin C, 800 IU (800 mg) vitamin E, 30 mg zinc, 60 mcg selenium, 4 mg copper, and 6 mg manganese. I take two fish oil capsules (1,000 mg each) each morning and one enteric-coated aspirin (325 mg) (easier on the stomach) each morning. Recently I have been taking 50 mg Pyc-nogenol. Also, since September 1995 I have taken 1.5 mg of mela-tonin almost nightly. (See Chapter 13, "Melatonin Update," for more information.)

Finally, I practice the other health-promoting habits recommended in this chapter. While Gay, my wife, may have some reservations about my driving, I always wear a seat belt. In the past I used to enjoy an occasional cigar but have not smoked one for ten years. I guard my sleep carefully and catch up on weekends if required. My family and I take at least one week of vacation yearly, and I usually take another two weeks of time away from work for travel (Australia, Sweden, China, and Holland in the past eighteen months). At least quarterly, I get away for a long weekend with Gay (San Diego last spring) or the grandchildren (Thanksgiving in Kansas with all my family and Gay's family). Finally, I exercise moderation in other areas, including alcohol use and work.

These are the health habits I recommend and practice myself. They are not awesomely time-consuming or unbearably difficult to incorporate into a planned but busy life. With these habits I feel good, have great energy, and enjoy very good health.

GENERAL PREVENTION— TAILORED PROTECTION—DISEASE REVERSAL

Hardening of the arteries can be reversed, tumors can shrink, and aging can be slowed. This antioxidant program kicks in at whatever stage you are, holds the line, and works on restoring health. Hazel (see Chapter 2) continues to outwit the aging process and surprise and amaze her relatives and friends. Robert (see Chapter 3) had a heart attack eight years ago but has no evidence of heart disease today. Marcie (see Chapter 7) had a breast cancer removed two years ago and has no evidence of cancer today.

Because you, our readers, are at different stages and at different risk levels, we developed three levels of intensity for this program. Because you have shown the interest to read this far, we call this your antioxidant, antiaging program. The general prevention program is designed for all adults and outlines the basic health-promoting steps that medical research indicates every adult should follow. See Table 8.1 and note the left-hand column.

TABLE 8.1   OUR ANTIOXIDANT, ANTIAGING PLAN*

ELEMENT	GENERAL PREVENTION ALL PEOPLE	TAILORED PROTECTION FOR ALL AT-RISK	DISEASE REVERSAL FOR PERSONS WITH SPECIFIED DISEASES
Diet			
Dietary fiber (C, H)	20–35 g daily	20–35 g/d; soluble fiber to normalize LDL chol.	20–35 g/d; soluble fiber to normalize LDL chol.
Vegetables + fruits (A,C,H)	3 + 2 servings per day	3 + 2 servings per day	3 + 2 servings per day
Fat intake (C,H)	<30% of calories	<25% of calories	<20% of calories
Fish (H)	2 servings fish weekly	2 servings fish weekly	2 servings fish weekly
Soy protein (C,H)	1 serving daily	2 servings daily	3 servings daily
Garlic (H)	Optional	4 times weekly	Daily
Green tea (A,C,H)	Daily	2 cups daily	2 cups daily
Nuts (H)	4 times weekly	4 times weekly	4 times weekly
Purple grapes (A,C,H)	Once daily	Twice daily	Twice daily
Vegetable juice (A,C,H)	12 oz. per day	12 oz. per day	12 oz. per day
Exercise			
Walking (A,C,H)	10 miles weekly	14 miles weekly	14 miles weekly
Upper body (H)	40 minutes weekly	70 minutes weekly	70 minutes weekly
Supplements			
Vitamin-mineral (A,C,H)	1 daily	1 daily	1 daily
BCES (A, C, H)	1 twice daily	2 twice daily	2 twice daily
Fish oil (H)	Optional	2 capsules daily for H	2 capsules daily for H
FABB (H)	Optional[†]	Optional[†]	Recommended for H
Aspirin (C, H)	1 daily	1 daily	1 daily
Melatonin (A)	Optional	Optional Recommended for A	Optional Recommended for A
Pycnogenol (A,C,H)	Optional	Optional Recommended for C	50 mg per day Recommended for C

Other

Nonsmoking (A,C,H)	Important	Essential	Vital
Seat belts	Important	Important	Important
Rest and relaxation (A,H)	Important	Important	Vital
Moderation (A,C,H)	Important	Important	Vital

* A = antiaging; C = cancer; H = heart disease.
† Daily intake of folic acid, vitamins B$_6$ and B$_{12}$ (FABB) recommended if you have a strong family history of early heart disease or developed early heart disease yourself (see Chapter 3).

TABLE 8.1.1   VITAMIN RECOMMENDED DAILY INTAKE, YOUR ANTIOXIDANT, ANTIAGING PLAN

VITAMIN	GENERAL PREVENTION	TAILORED PROTECTION	DISEASE REVERSAL
Beta-carotene	6 mg (10,000 IU)	12 mg (20,000 IU)	12 mg (20,000 IU)
Vitamin C	250 mg twice daily	500 mg twice daily	500 mg twice daily
Vitamin E	400 mg (400 IU)	800 mg (800 IU)	800 mg (800 IU)

The tailored protection program is designed for persons at higher risk for aging, cancer, or heart disease. This applies to persons who have a family history of Alzheimer's disease, a strong family history of breast or colon cancer, or early heart attacks in the family. This also applies to persons who have risk factors such as cigarette smoking, high blood pressure, blood fat abnormalities (see Chapter 3), diabetes, obesity, low levels of physical activity, or poor stress management techniques. We recommend that these individuals start at the general prevention level for diet and exercise. We also recommend that persons in this category begin taking supplements at the midrange level (see Table 8.1.1) and that they stop smoking as soon as possible. If you smoke and are unable to stop, we recommend that you move to the highest level of protection, as indicated in the disease reversal column (Table 8.1.1).

The disease reversal level of the program is designed for persons who have established disease. Thus, if you have a history of cancer of any type (except skin cancer related to excessive sun exposure), we recommend you embark on this program. This applies if you have blood circulation problems, including a previous heart attack, a history of angina pectoris (chest pain related to the heart), a previous stroke or transient ischemic attacks (also called TIAs), or poor circulation to the legs. If you have had X rays that show blockage or major narrowing of blood vessels to the heart, brain, or legs, you should strive to achieve the guidelines in the right-hand column of Table 8.1. *We recommend you start on the diet and exercise recommendations in the general prevention section and gradually, over several months, move to the tailored protection and then to the disease reversal level. For supplements, start at the disease reversal level immediately.* Examine your rest, relaxation, and moderation practices and see how they match the recommendations. You may need to have a family member or friend give you a more objective opinion about how your lifestyle matches these guidelines before assuming that you are doing well in these areas.

YOUR ANTIOXIDANT, ANTIAGING PROGRAM

Central to your antioxidant food program is the intake of vegetables and fruits rich in antioxidants. Vegetables such as broccoli, carrots, and spinach; sweet potatoes; and fruits such as apricots, cantaloupe, kiwi, and oranges are rich in antioxidant vitamins and also in other phytochemicals that protect you from developing cancer. While antioxidant supplements offer health protection, intake of these vital vegetables and fruits provides Mother Nature's most protective phytochemicals tailored to reduce your risks of premature aging, cancer, and heart disease. Your program is designed to help you gradually incorporate these foods into your daily eating plan so that you are receiving optimal protection from all these conditions.

Table 8.1 gives you a bird's-eye view of the food, exercise, supplement, and other elements that make up your comprehensive antioxidant program. We first will focus on the food part. Table 8.2 lists vegetables and fruits that have high levels of the antioxidant vitamins beta-carotene and vitamin C. In Appendix Table B you can find a detailed list of the antioxidant vitamin contents of commonly used vegetables and fruits. While we highlight the vegetables and fruits rich in antioxidant vitamins, this does not tell the whole story. Many studies indicate that broccoli and other cruciferous vegetables protect from developing various forms of cancer. Also, garlic and onions offer major health benefits with respect to reducing risk for heart disease and cancer. The health benefits of soy protein products and the important isoflavones contained in soy products are summarized in Chapter 7.

TABLE 8.2   HONOR ROLL OF VEGETABLES AND FRUITS

The top section includes foods rich in both beta-carotene and vitamin C. These foods are selected because they provide, on average, more than 50 percent of the daily recommended intake for these important antioxidants. Other health-promoting vegetables and fruits are listed in the bottom section.

HIGH IN ANTIOXIDANTS

Vegetables
broccoli
carrots
red peppers
spinach
sweet potatoes
vegetable juice

Fruits
apricots
cantaloupe
grapefruit
kiwi
oranges

OTHER HEALTH BENEFITS

cruciferous vegetables
   (broccoli, Brussels
sprouts, cabbage,
cauliflower, radishes,
turnips, watercress—
rich in healthful
phytochemicals)
allium vegetables
   (garlic, onions,
scallions—rich in
sulfur-containing
healthful phytochemicals)

bananas (high in potassium)
grapes (rich in polyphenols)

soy protein products
  (isolated soy protein,
soy flour, soy beverage,
textured soy protein, tofu)

Table 8.3 is a worksheet you can use to make your plan for increasing your use of these specific health-promoting vegetables and fruits. Do this one meal at a time. For example, start with breakfast. Can you start drinking hot tea and either drinking juice or eating fruit from the recommended list? You can do that, can't you? Right! After two weeks you will be having an antioxidant-rich, health-promoting breakfast.

TABLE 8.3 WORKSHEET FOR INCREASING YOUR INTAKE OF ANTIOXIDANT-RICH FOODS

Meal	Suggestions	Dr. Anderson's Favorites	Your Favorites
Breakfast			
Beverage	Hot tea (nonherbal)	Green tea	
Juice	Grape, grapefruit, orange, V-8	Grape (occasionally)	
Fruit	Cantaloupe, oranges, grapefruit	Banana	
Cereal	Oatmeal, oat bran	Oatmeal	
Lunch			
Beverage	V-8 juice or iced tea	V-8 juice	
Vegetables	Carrots, broccoli, spinach salad	Broccoli, carrots, red peppers	
Bread	Whole grain bread or crackers	Banana-nut soy muffins	
Sandwich filling	Turkey or low-fat choice	None	
Fruit	Apricots, grapes, oranges	Grapes or oranges	

Meal	Suggestions	Dr. Anderson's Favorites	Your Favorites
Evening meal			
Beverage	Iced tea, hot tea, V-8 or grape juice	Iced tea or V-8 juice	
Salad	Spinach or dark greens, shredded carrots, low-fat dressing	Large vegetable salad, ½ oz. pecans, low-fat dressing	
Entrée	Soy protein entrée, bean burrito, fish, lean meat or poultry	Vegetable-tofu stir-fry (includes garlic)	
Vegetables	Broccoli, carrots, red peppers, spinach, sweet potatoes, vegetable juice	Sweet potatoes	
Fruit (dessert: special occasions)	Apricots, bananas, cantaloupe, grapefruit, grapes, kiwi, oranges	Mixed fruit, 2 cups (kiwi, oranges, melon) (fig cookies)	

Look at lunch. If you take your lunch you can put in a vegetable juice and a fruit. Make sure your other choices are low-fat. If you eat out, choose iced tea or orange juice. Have a piece of fruit or a fruit cup for the final item. Try a large salad with a low-fat dressing and low-fat crackers as the main choice. If you pack your lunch you can put in carrot sticks, broccoli, celery, and strips of red peppers. Buy some baby carrots and have them for lunch or for munchies.

At dinner, focus on identifying entrées that are antioxidant-rich. Any soy protein product will fit the bill. You may be like a friend from New Jersey who said: "I've heard of tofu but don't know what it is." If so, you may want to start with items such as taco fillings, sloppy joes, and chili made from textured soy protein (see the recipes in Chapter 9). Try some of our soy muffins. As you grow fond of soy, try the vegetable stir-fry recipes in Chapter 9. After you

TABLE 8.4 MENU PLANS

MEAL OR NUTRIENT	DAY 1	DAY 2	DAY 3	DAY 4	DAY 5
BREAKFAST	Vegetable juice, 1 cup Allison's French Toast 1 serving* Pancake syrup, 2 tbsp Strawberries, 1/2 cup Green tea, 2 cups	Tangy vegetable juice, 1 serving* Banana-Nut Soy muffins, 2* Sunny Fruit Fiesta, 1 serving* Green tea, 2 cups	Grapefruit, 1/2 Apple Soy Muffins, 2* Skim milk, 1/2 cup Green tea, 2 cups	Sunny Fruit Fiesta, 1 serving* English muffin, 1 Fat-free cream cheese, 1 tbsp Green tea, 2 cups	Orange juice, 1/2 cup Oat meal, 2/3 cup Skim milk, 1/2 cup Apricots, dried, 1/4 cup Whole wheat bread, 1 slice Green tea, 2 cups
LUNCH	Turkey sandwich: whole wheat bread, 2 slices; turkey, 2 oz; tomato; lettuce; mustard Three-bean salad, 1 cup Carrots, 1/2 cup Celery, 1/2 cup Grapes, 1/2 cup Iced tea	Pita bread sandwich: 1 whole wheat pita bread; tuna salad, low-fat dressing Broccoli, 1 cup Banana, 1 Sparkling water	Pasta salad: Spaghetti, cooked, 1/2 cup Chickpeas, cooked 2 oz Onions, carrots, broccoli Fat-free Italian dressing Kiwifruit, 1 Diet cola	Vegetable juice, 12 oz Broccoli, 1 cup with Sour cream, 2 tbsp Super-Easy Your Choice Muffins, 2* Mandarin oranges, 1/2 cup Iced tea	Down Home Chili, 1 serving* Carrots, 1/2 cup Celery, 1/2 cup Saltine crackers, 5 Diet soda

DINNER	*Spinach salad:* spinach; tomatoes; onion; fat-free Italian dressing Bread sticks, 2 olive oil, 1/3 tbsp garlic powder Red pepper spaghetti, 1 serving* Citrus surprise, 1 serving* Iced tea	Won-ton soup, 4 oz Sweet and Sour Tofu, 1 serving* White rice, 1 cup Iced tea	Tortilla chips, low fat, 5 Bean dip, fat-free, 2 tbsp *Vegetarian tacos** Spanish rice, 1/2 cup Iceberg lettuce salad with tomatoes, onions, Fat-free Catalina dressing, Low-fat cheese, 1 oz Tutti-frutti, 1 serving* Iced tea	Citrus Spinach Salad, 1 serving* Soy Good Pizza, 1 serving* Banana, 1 Sparkling water	Tangy Vegetable Juice, 1 serving* Gazpacho, 1 serving* Whitefish, broiled, 4 oz Tofu Sweet Potato Bake, 1 serving* Turnip greens, boiled, 1/2 cup Dinner roll, 1 Sparkling water
SNACK	Oat bran cold cereal, 1/2 cup Skim milk, 1 cup	Thin twisted pretzels, 10 Skim milk, 1/2 cup	Apricot Pumpkin Bread, 1 serving* Sparkling water	Raisin bread, 1 slice Skim milk, 1/2 cup Decaffeinated tea	Strawberry-Banana Frosty, 1 serving* Cinnamon-raisin bagel, 1/2
CALORIES	1589	1608	1626	1589	1592
SOY PROTEIN, G	8	11	25	9	21
BETA-CAROTENE, MG	5	4	1	1	6
VITAMIN C, MG	332	378	212	535	399

*Recipes for these items are in Chapter 9.

have gotten into the antioxidant main dish, the rest of the evening meal is easy to modify.

To complement the main dish, start with a salad rich in antioxidant vegetables. Spinach and other dark green leafy vegetables are your best choices. You can spice up the salad with pecans or walnuts. Be sure to use either a low-fat dressing or small amounts of olive oil. For a beverage, try iced tea or use vegetable or grape juice as an appetizer. Red wine can be substituted for grape juice, if you prefer, and still give you the important antioxidant polyphenols originating from the grape. Eat at least two different vegetables on the side. Try to have one serving of cruciferous vegetables (see Table 8.3) and one serving of beta-carotene-rich vegetables (carrots, sweet potatoes, or vegetable juice) (see Table 8.3) each evening. To finish the meal, choose from some of the fruits recommended in Table 8.2 or Table 8.3. Fresh fruit in a salad is the most nutritious and tasty, but canned fruit also fits the bill. Apricots, grapefruit sections, and mandarin oranges are good choices. You can enhance these by cutting up a fresh kiwi to add color and flavor.

Most people will need six weeks to make these changes in their diet. As outlined above, my diet has evolved over eighteen years and still is changing. I incorporated soy products into my diet over a two-week period and switched to antioxidant-rich vegetables and fruits over a four-week period. So don't try to do all of this overnight.

Table 8.4 provides a 5-day menu plan for a 1600 calorie intake. This illustrates the great variety of food provided on the antioxidant-antiaging program and shows how you can incorporate more soy protein, beta-carotene and vitamin C into your daily eating habits.

YOUR ANTIOXIDANT, ANTIAGING EXERCISE PROGRAM

Chapter 10 outlines the exercise program and the health benefits of regular exercise. Remember that the health benefits start with walking six miles per week and increase at twelve, twenty, and thirty-five miles per week. Twelve miles of walking per week greatly reduces your risks of cancer, heart attack, and premature aging. Doing aerobic exercises using the upper arms (such as swimming or cross-country skiing) improves health and increases cardiovascular fitness. As Table 8.1 summarizes, we recommend a cross-training program involving walking at least ten miles per week and using an aerobic upper-body exercise under aerobic conditions for ten minutes four times weekly.

YOUR ANTIOXIDANT, ANTIAGING SUPPLEMENT PROGRAM

Recently an expert panel met in Washington, DC, to make recommendations to the FDA about antioxidant supplement recommendations. After two days of deliberation, the panel developed a consensus that health agencies should not recommend use of antioxidant supplements by healthy adults or even adults at high risk for cancer or heart disease or with established heart disease. These experts used these lines of reasoning: First, although the evidence from population studies and other studies is compelling, there have not been prospective clinical trials documenting that antioxidant supplement use reduces risk of cancer or heart disease. (The study from China described in Chapter 4 was not persuasive, in their opinion, and needs to be confirmed.). Second, although there appear to be no side effects or risks for the commonly recommended doses, the long-term safety of these doses has not been documented. Third, the panel was concerned that people would take a supplement capsule instead of eating less fat or stopping smoking.

After this prestigious panel made these recommendations, someone in the audience asked the panel members whether they personally took antioxidant supplements. About 75 percent of the panel sheepishly held up their hands. Later, in private, one of the panel members confided: "From what I know about antioxidants, I would be stupid not to take supplements myself." Thus the recommendations that we make (see Table 8.1.1) are controversial. Some feel that antioxidant supplements should not be recommended to the general public. Many experts, however, take the supplements themselves. Based on our research and the information summarized in this book, we feel that the benefits of taking antioxidant supplements far outweigh the risks. Thus we feel strongly that you will benefit from taking the supplements at the levels outlined in Table 8.1.1.

MULTIPLE VITAMIN-MINERAL SUPPLEMENTS

Because it is difficult to obtain the variety of foods each day to get all the recommended amounts of vitamins and minerals, we recommend that all adults take a "once a day" capsule without iron. If you have anemia or heavy menstrual periods, your doctor may recommend that you take an iron supplement. However, most men and postmenopausal women do not need additional iron. Iron is a prooxidant that promotes the generation of free radicals, so don't take iron unless your doctor recommends it. Take the supplement with or immediately after a meal.

To avoid osteoporosis, each American adult should take a calcium supplement. These recommendations grow out of the recommendations for daily calcium intake of the Consensus Panel of the National Institutes of Health. Women aged twenty-five to fifty and men aged twenty-five to sixty-five years should take a supplement of 500 mg per day. Women over age fifty and men over sixty-five years should take 1,000 mg per day. These supplements should usually be calcium carbonate tablets. Buy the least expensive form of calcium carbonate, and daily take at least 500 mg or 1,000 mg of elemental calcium (that means 500 mg or 1,000 mg of calcium rather than a 500 mg tablet of calcium carbonate). Take one tablet with or immediately after breakfast and, if required, one tablet with or immediately after dinner.

ANTIOXIDANT SUPPLEMENTS

We recommend that all adults take a combination of beta-carotene (10,000 to 20,000 IU or 6 to 12 mg daily), vitamin C (250 to 500 mg twice daily), and vitamin E (400 IU or 400 mg daily). For tailored protection or disease reversal, you should take twice this amount. Combination capsules are widely available that provide these levels of antioxidant vitamins. Popular brand names include Protegra, Procea, and Vitegra. Most of these contain selenium, zinc, copper, and manganese. As stated above, I take four capsules daily. Take antioxidant capsules with breakfast or dinner or immediately afterward. Always drink 8 ounces of water or fluid after taking these tablets or capsules.

FISH OIL

Fish oil capsules, rich in a special type of fatty acids called omega-3 fatty acids, act to decrease serum triglycerides. Eating fish twice weekly is associated with a lower rate of heart disease than only occasional intake of fish. If your blood triglycerides are elevated, intake of two fish oil capsules may lower these levels. Perhaps the intake of fish oil capsules reduces risk of heart attack by decreasing blood clot formation. If you are unable to eat fish twice weekly, you might hedge your bets by taking fish oil capsules. Take these capsules with or immediately after meals.

FOLIC ACID AND VITAMINS B$_6$ AND B$_{12}$ (FABB)

As discussed in Chapter 3, high blood levels of homocysteine, an amino acid or protein building block, may contribute to premature heart attacks. If family members have had heart attacks before age fifty, you may want to protect yourself by taking these vitamins. Research indicates that use of these vitamins significantly decreases blood homocysteine levels (see Glossary, Appendix C). For protection from these problems the recommended levels of vitamins daily are these: folic acid, 1 mg; vitamin B$_6$, 50 mg; and vitamin B$_{12}$, 10 mcg. These tablets can be taken before or after meals.

ASPIRIN

Dozens of studies indicate that intake of aspirin decreases risk of heart attack. Regular intake of aspirin decreases the aggregation or clumping of platelets and decreases formation of blood clots. Recent evidence indicates that regular intake of aspirin decreases risk of colon cancer. We recommend one enteric-coated aspirin (325 mg) per day. The orange, enteric coating protects the stomach from the ulcer-producing potential of aspirin. Take after meals.

MELATONIN

This hormone is primarily produced by the pineal gland, the "master gland" in the center of the brain. The pineal gland works as a "pacemaker" for the entire body and also serves as our "biological clock." Much of the regulation of body rhythms is accomplished by the release of melatonin, a peptide (containing amino acids) hormone. In addition to its being produced and released by the pineal gland, recent research indicates that this hormone is produced in many other cells of the body.[1] Other recent research indicates that melatonin is a potent antioxidant.[2]

Melatonin's chief claim to fame is as an "antiaging hormone." In young children, melatonin blood levels are very high, about 350 units per 100 ml, but levels decrease dramatically as we age, to about 30 units per 100 ml by age ninety.[3] Persons with Alzheimer's disease have very low levels of melatonin, and some researchers suggest that the low levels of hormone allow the brain cells to be damaged by free radicals. In certain animal models of aging, administration of melatonin has had dramatic effects in slowing this aging process. See Chapter 13, "Melatonin Update," for further information.[1, 4, 5]

PYCNOGENOL

This group of phytochemicals, contained in a patented product, contain subtonics called proanthocyanidins (PACs), which are extracted from the bark of certain pine trees and/or from grape seeds. Because they are water-soluble and have vitamin C-like antioxidant effects, they have been called "vitamin C helpers."[6] Since they are in the fibrous part of fruits and vegetables, much of which is discarded, and since much of the fiber is poorly digested, the PAC chemicals contained within may not be fully absorbed. Yet these substances may have special protective properties, including reducing risks for blood vessel diseases and diabetic retinopathy (eye disease).[6] As summarized by Passwater and Kandaswami,[6] the PACs may slow the aging process, reduce risk for several forms of cancer, and protect from heart attack. Further research is required to confirm these possibilities. Since Pycnogenol is produced by a patented process and since it contains a mixture of bioflavonoids,[6] it can be fairly expensive. Nevertheless, because of its potential benefit as a potent phytochemical and antioxidant, Dr. Anderson recommends a daily intake of 50 mg for persons in the disease reversal category (see Table 8.1).

OTHER HEALTH-PROMOTING HABITS

NONSMOKING

Currently about 46 million Americans smoke. Smoking causes approximately 420,000 deaths per year, second only to cardiovascular disease, and costs an estimated $47 billion for direct and indirect costs. Cigarette smoking causes or contributes to development of these health problems: lung cancer and a variety of other cancers; lung disease, including bronchitis, emphysema, and pneumonia;

coronary heart disease, stroke, and other problems with hardening of the arteries; cataracts; infertility, stillbirths, and premature births; and osteoporosis.[7] Perhaps 5 to 10 percent of cigarette smokers, in my estimation, have chronic anxiety disorders that almost preclude them from stopping smoking. However, most smokers can stop if they make a firm commitment to do so. In my previous book[8] we provide specific guidelines for helping people stop smoking.

SEAT BELTS

Some experts estimate that the uniform use of seat belts would save 30,000 lives annually in the United States. If you buckle your seat belt every time you are in an automobile, you will reduce your estimated risk for serious injury or death by more than 50 percent. It's worth the extra money for the protection offered by dual airbags.

REST AND RELAXATION

Important for health and longevity are these behaviors:

- getting adequate sleep, and feeling rested when you get up in the morning;
- spending quality nonworking time with family and friends;
- having weekend escapes several times yearly;
- taking at least one week of peaceful and relaxing vacation per year.

In my previous books I give more details on what you should do and how you *can* do it.[7,8]

MODERATION

To further enhance your health and longevity, follow these guidelines:

- Don't smoke.
- Abstain from alcohol, or use it moderately (one glass of red wine daily for women and two glasses for men).
- Don't use sleeping pills, tranquilizers, or antidepressants unless your doctor strongly feels that you need them. Try cutting down or avoiding caffeine and use relaxation techniques to help with your sleep; give melatonin a try.
- Don't be a workaholic (not many people have the deathbed complaint "I wish I had spent more time in the office").

In my two previous books I write in more detail about these topics.[7, 8]

TO SUM UP

YOUR ANTIOXIDANT FOOD PLAN

- Among vegetables, seek out these that are rich in antioxidants and have several servings daily: broccoli, carrots, red peppers, spinach, sweet potatoes, and vegetable juice. Include other cruciferous vegetables (such as cabbage, cauliflower, and radishes) and garlic or onions.
- Among fruits, include daily some of these that are rich in antioxidants: apricots, cantaloupe, grapefruit, kiwi, and oranges. Also eat bananas and grapes as often as possible.
- Eat foods high in fiber (20 to 35 g daily) and low in fat (fewer than 30 percent of your total calories), or even lower for people at high risk).
- Enjoy soy protein—at least seven servings per week, or even more if needed.
- Drink green tea, hot or iced. Black tea or other nonherbal tea may provide the same benefits. Drink two to three cups or glasses per day.

FRUITS AND VEGETABLES PROVIDE ELIXIR FOR LONG LIFE

Spanish explorer Ponce de León came closer to finding the fountain of youth than he realized. From Indians in Puerto Rico he had heard tales of an island that reputedly possessed a magic fountain, a spring whose water had the power to restore youth. Searching for this legendary fountain, he discovered Florida in 1513. Twenty-six years later, the fountain of youth still had not been discovered, but another Spanish explorer, Hernando de Soto, reported that Florida Indians had plentiful supplies of "pumpkins and other vegetables"—rich sources of life-prolonging beta-carotene and other antioxidants. Ironically, it was another Spaniard, Pedro Menéndez de Avilés, who brought a real youth elixir to America. In the year 1565 he planted oranges in Florida. Oranges, a prime source of the antioxidant vitamin C, can help postpone the ravages of old age. In fact, an overwhelming amount of research indicates that consumption of antioxidant vitamins C, E, and beta-carotene strengthens our immune systems and reduces our risks of cancer, cardiovascular problems, and other degenerative diseases.

EXERCISE

- Walk at least ten miles per week, more if you have risk factors or heart disease.
- Do forty minutes of aerobic, upper-body exercise (a machine known as an E-force cross-trainer is effective) or more weekly.

SUPPLEMENTS

- Take one multiple vitamin-mineral supplement daily.
- Include two to four antioxidant supplements daily to include at least 10,000 IU of beta-carotene, 500 mg of vitamin C, and 400 IU of vitamin E.
- Take one enteric-coated aspirin daily.

- Optional recommendations:

    fish oil capsules—two daily for high triglyceride level or heart disease;

    FABB (folic acid, vitamins B_6 and B_{12}) as directed;

    melatonin—for sleep, jet lag, or Alzheimer's disease prophylactic use;

    Pycnogenol—optional for potential prevention of aging, cancer, diabetic complications, and heart disease.

9

WONDERFUL ANTIOXIDANT ANTIAGING RECIPES

BREAKFAST

ALLISON'S NEW FRENCH TOAST

1 cup (8 oz) unflavored soy
  beverage
½ cup (4 oz) egg substitute
½ tsp vanilla

1 tbsp brown sugar
  Cinnamon
8 thick slices white bread

Mix first 4 ingredients together and pour into shallow bowl. Spray skillet or griddle with canola nonstick cooking spray and heat. Dip bread in liquid mixture one piece at a time, coating both sides. Place in skillet and sprinkle liberally with cinnamon; grill each side until golden brown and crispy, about 5 to 7 minutes. Serves 4.

Serve hot with mashed blueberries, mashed strawberries, or maple syrup.

Nutrients per serving

Calories: 204	Carbohydrates: 32 g	Protein: 10 g
Saturated fat: 1 g	Monounsaturated fat: 1 g	Cholesterol: 0
Fiber: 1 g	Soy protein: 3 g	Fat: 4 g

Comment: Our oldest granddaughter, age six years, and her grand-dad make this for the family on Saturday mornings.

APPLE PANCAKES

1 cup all-purpose flour	2 tsp baking powder
1/4 cup soy flour	1 1/4 cup soy milk (beverage)
3 tbsp sugar	1/4 cup (2 oz) egg substitute
1/2 tsp cinnamon	1 tsp vanilla extract
1/4 tsp nutmeg	1 tart apple peeled, cored, and
1/8 tsp salt	grated

Mix the first 7 dry ingredients. In a separate bowl, blend together the milk, egg substitute, and vanilla extract. Pour liquid ingredients over dry ingredients and blend together. Fold in the apples. Spray griddle or skillet with canola cooking spray and heat. Pour 1/4 cupfuls of batter onto medium-hot griddle. Heat for 2 minutes or until bubbles appear on surface. Flip and cook for another minute or until heated through. Served topped with applesauce and maple syrup. Makes 12 pancakes to serve 4.

Nutrients per serving

Calories: 252	Carbohydrates: 46 g	Protein: 10 g
Saturated fat: 0	Monounsaturated fat: 0	Cholesterol: 0
Fiber: 1 g	Soy protein: 5 g	Fat: 3 g

SUNNY FRUIT FIESTA

1 cantaloupe melon, halved and seeded	1 1/2 tsp lime peel, grated (optional)
1/4 cup granulated sugar	2 kiwi fruit, peeled and sliced
1/4 cup lime juice	1 cup purple grapes
2 tbsp lemon juice	1 cup mandarin orange sections

Using a melon baller, scoop flesh from cantaloupe into balls and set aside. Into a large glass bowl combine the sugar, lime juice, lemon juice, and lime peel. Stir well to dissolve sugar. Add the melon balls, kiwi, grapes, and mandarin orange slices. Toss gently to combine. Cover bowl with plastic wrap and refrigerate for at least 1 hour to blend flavors, stirring once or twice. Spoon the fruit into serving bowls, dividing evenly. Serve immediately. Serves 4.

Nutrients per serving

Calories: 120	Carbohydrates: 31 g	Protein: 2 g
Saturated fat: 0	Monounsaturated fat: 0	Cholesterol: 0
Fiber: 3 g	Vitamin C: 87 mg	Fat: 0

BREAKFAST OR SNACK TIME

APPLE SOY MUFFINS

1½ cups enriched flour	¼ tsp nutmeg
½ cup soy flour	½ cup unflavored soy beverage
½ cup brown sugar	½ cup (4 oz) egg substitute
1 tbsp baking powder	2 tbsp canola oil
⅛ tsp salt	1 tsp vanilla
1 tsp cinnamon	1½ apples, shredded

Heat oven to 400°F. Spray twelve 2½-inch muffin pan cups with canola cooking spray. Combine dry ingredients (flour, sugar, baking powder, salt, cinnamon, and nutmeg) in a large bowl. Whisk wet ingredients (soy beverage, egg substitute, oil, and vanilla) together. Stir apples into dry ingredients until coated. Add wet ingredients to apples and dry ingredients and stir until just combined. Do not overstir.

Spoon into pan cups and bake for 20 minutes or until toothpick inserted into center comes out clean. Cool in pan for 5 minutes. Remove from pan and serve. Makes 12 muffins.

Nutrients per serving

Calories: 156	Carbohydrates: 26 g	Protein: 5 g
Saturated fat: 0	Monounsaturated fat: 2 g	Cholesterol: 0
Fiber: 1 g	Soy protein: 2 g	Fat: 4 g

APRICOT PUMPKIN BREAD

1 cup all-purpose flour	¼ tsp ginger
¾ cup soy flour	1 cup granulated sugar
1 tsp baking soda	½ cup dried apricots, chopped
½ tsp salt	½ cup (4 oz) egg substitute
1 tsp cinnamon	2 tbsp canola oil
½ tsp ground cloves	⅓ cup water
¼ tsp nutmeg	1 15 oz can pumpkin

Preheat oven to 350°F. Sift flour and add dry ingredients, including apricots and mix.

Mix egg substitute, oil, water, and pumpkin. Combine pumpkin mixture with dry ingredients and stir until blended. Pour into baking tin and bake at 350°F for 40–50 minutes or until a toothpick comes out clean when inserted into the center. Serves 12.

Nutrients per serving

Calories: 190	Carbohydrates: 34 g	Protein: 5 g
Saturated fat: 0	Monounsaturated fat: 2 g	Cholesterol: 0
Fiber: 2 g	Soy protein: 2 g	Fat: 4 g

Comment: Belinda brought this tasty bread to staff meeting and it received rave reviews from our staff which includes some finicky eaters.

Banana Nut Soy Muffins

1½ cups enriched flour
½ cup soy flour
½ cup brown sugar
1 tbsp baking powder
⅛ tsp salt
1 tsp cinnamon
1 cup unflavored soy beverage

½ cup (4 oz) egg substitute
2 tbsp canola oil
1 tsp vanilla
1 ripe banana, diced
½ cup raisins or chopped walnuts

Heat oven to 400°F. Spray 12 2½-inch muffin pan cups with canola cooking spray.

Combine dry ingredients (flour, sugar, baking powder, salt, and nutmeg) in a large bowl.

Whisk wet ingredients (soy beverage, egg substitute, oil, and vanilla) together. Stir bananas and raisins or walnuts into dry ingredients until coated. Stir in wet ingredients until just combined; do not overstir.

Spoon into pan cups and bake for 20 minutes or until toothpick inserted into center comes out clean. Cool in pan for 5 minutes. Remove from pan and serve. Makes 12 muffins.

Nutrients per serving

Calories: 182
Saturated fat: 0
Fiber: 1 g

Carbohydrates: 31 g
Monounsaturated fat: 2 g
Soy protein: 2 g

Protein: 5 g
Cholesterol: 0
Fat: 4 g

Comment: Jim served these at a press conference in August 1995 and received favorable comments from a number of media people, including a rather picky medical television personality.

BLUEBERRY SOY MUFFINS

1 cup blueberries, washed and drained
1½ cups enriched flour
½ cup soy flour
¼ cup brown sugar
1 tsp baking powder

½ tsp baking soda
⅛ tsp salt
½ cup unflavored soy beverage
½ cup (4 oz) egg substitute
1 tbsp canola oil
2 tsp liquid butter substitute

Heat oven to 375°F. Spray 12 2½-inch muffin pan cups with canola cooking spray.

Combine dry ingredients (flour, sugar, baking powder, baking soda, salt) in a large bowl.

Whisk wet ingredients (soy beverage, egg substitute, and oil) together.

Stir blueberries into dry ingredients until coated. Stir wet ingredients into blueberries and dry ingredients until just combined; do not overstir.

Spoon into pan cups and bake for 20 minutes or until toothpick inserted into center comes out clean. Cool in pan for 5 minutes. Remove from pan and serve. Makes 12 muffins.

Nutrients per serving

Calories: 130
Saturated fat: 0
Fiber: 1 g

Carbohydrates: 20 g
Monounsaturated fat: 1 g
Soy protein: 2 g

Protein: 5 g
Cholesterol: 0
Fat: 3 g

SUPER-EASY YOUR-CHOICE MUFFINS

1 7-oz package muffin mix   ⅓ cup soy flour
   (banana nut, blueberry,   ½ cup (4 oz) unflavored soy
   blackberry, oat bran, etc.)   milk (beverage)

Spray muffin tin with canola cooking spray. Mix muffin mix and flour. Add soy milk and stir until dry ingredients are moist; do not mix. Fill 6 muffin tins about ⅔ full. Bake for 10 to 12 minutes at 375°F in a preheated oven or as instructed on the package until muffins are lightly brown or spring back when touched. Makes 6 muffins.

Nutrients per serving

Calories: 155   Carbohydrates: 24 g   Protein: 4 g
Saturated fat: 1 g   Monounsaturated fat: 2 g   Cholesterol: 0
Fiber: 1 g   Soy protein: 3 g   Fat: 5 g

Comment: Another very simple breakfast or snack. Jim makes these to take to Sunday evening church committee meetings to keep everyone happy and focused. For a group, you can get the minimuffin tins and make 10 muffins instead of 6.

LUNCH OR DINNER DISHES

SALADS

CITRUS SPINACH SALAD

6 cups torn fresh spinach
(8 oz)
2 large oranges, cut into thin
slices and halved
1 cup sliced fresh mushrooms
1 tbsp lemon juice

1 tbsp canola oil
1 tbsp water
1/2 tsp poppy seeds
1/4 tsp salt
1 ripe avocado cut into long
slices (optional)

Prepare spinach, orange slices, and mushrooms; cover and chill. In a screw-top jar combine lemon juice, oil, water, poppy seeds, and salt; cover and shake well; chill. Arrange spinach, orange slices, mushroom slices, and avocado on salad plate. Shake again and pour the dressing over the salad. Serve immediately. Serves 6.

Nutrients per serving

Calories: 62	Carbohydrates: 9 g	Protein: 2 g
Saturated fat: 0	Monounsaturated fat: 1 g	Cholesterol: 0
Fiber: 2 g	Vitamin C: 39 mg	Fat: 2 g

Comment: This is our favorite salad for company.

TOMATO-ONION SALAD

1/4 cup balsamic vinegar
3 tbsp water
1 tsp olive oil
1 tsp Dijon mustard
1/4 tsp black pepper
1/8 tsp salt

5 medium unpeeled tomatoes
1 large purple onion, thinly sliced and separated into rings
2 tsp minced fresh oregano

Combine first 6 ingredients in a jar; cover tightly and shake vigorously. Set aside. Core tomatoes and cut each into 6 slices. Layer tomatoes and onion slices in a shallow dish; sprinkle with oregano. Pour vinegar mixture over vegetables; cover and marinate in refrigerator 3 hours. Serves 8.

Nutrients per serving

Calories: 54   Carbohydrates: 8 g   Protein: 2 g
Saturated fat: 0   Monounsaturated fat: 1 g Cholesterol: 0
Fiber: 1 g   Fat: 2 g

SOUPS

GAZPACHO

2 tbsp lemon juice
2 cloves garlic, minced
1 tsp dry dill weed
1 slice day-old bread, crumbled
2 16-ounce cans stewed tomatoes
1 green pepper, chopped
5 green onions, chopped

1 medium cucumber, chopped
1/2 tsp salt (optional)
1 tsp sugar
1 10 1/2-oz can reduced-fat chicken broth
Tabasco (to taste)
Black pepper (to taste)

Process lemon juice, garlic, dill, and bread in blender until smooth. Add remaining ingredients and blend well. Season with Tabasco and pepper to taste. Chill for 4 to 5 hours. Serves 6.

Nutrients per serving

Calories: 92	Carbohydrates: 18 g	Protein: 4 g
Saturated fat: 0	Monounsaturated fat: 0	Cholesterol: 0
Fiber: 4 g	Vitamin C: 71 mg	Fat: 1 g

Comment: This tasty soup is a great way to start a meal.

CURRIED CARROT SOUP

6 medium carrots, thinly sliced	2 tsp curry powder
2 cups vegetable stock	½ cup unflavored soy milk
1 small onion, chopped	(beverage)

Combine all ingredients except the soy milk and cook over medium heat until carrots are tender. Pour into blender and puree until smooth. Stir in soy milk. Warm over low heat until hot. Serves 4.

Nutrients per serving

Calories: 96	Carbohydrates: 19 g	Protein: 3 g
Saturated fat: 0	Monounsaturated fat: 0	Cholesterol: 0
Fiber: 3 g	Soy protein: 1 g	Beta-carotene: 3 mg
Fat: 1 g		

CREAMY SPINACH SOUP

Nonstick spray
1 tsp canola oil
1 small onion, chopped
1 10¾-oz can of reduced-fat condensed cream of mushroom soup
1 soup can water

⅛ tsp ground nutmeg
⅛ tsp black pepper
1 10-oz package frozen chopped spinach
½ cup plain nonfat yogurt, divided
Red pepper strips (optional)

Spray 2-quart saucepan with cooking spray. Heat canola oil for 1 minute over medium heat. Add onion; cook until onion is tender, stirring constantly. Stir in soup, water, nutmeg, and pepper. Add spinach. Heat to boiling, breaking up spinach with fork and stirring occasionally. Reduce heat to low. Cover; cook 5 minutes or until spinach is tender. Remove from heat. In covered blender, blend half of soup mixture and ¼ cup yogurt until smooth. Pour into serving bowl. Repeat with remaining soup mixture and yogurt. Garnish with sweet red pepper strips if desired. Serves 4.

Nutrients per serving

Calories: 99	Carbohydrates: 13	Protein: 5 g
Saturated fat: 1 g	Monounsaturated fat: 1 g	Cholesterol: 7 mg
Fiber: 3 g	Vitamin C: 10 mg	Fat: 3 g

SPICY TOMATO-ONION

1 tbsp canola oil
2 cups chopped onions
2 tsp grated orange rind
5 cloves garlic, minced
1½ tsp ground cumin
1 tsp dried whole basil

1 tsp crushed red pepper
4 14½-oz cans stewed tomatoes, undrained and chopped
2 10½-oz cans low-sodium chicken broth

Heat oil in large saucepan over medium heat. Add onion, orange rind, and garlic and sauté 8 minutes until onion is tender. Add cumin, basil, and red pepper; sauté 1 minute. Add tomatoes and chicken broth; bring to a boil. Reduce heat and simmer, uncovered, 30 minutes. Serves 9.

Nutrients per serving

Calories: 87	Carbohydrates: 16 g	Protein: 3 g
Saturated fat: 0	Monounsaturated fat: 1 g	Cholesterol: 0
Fiber: 3 g	Vitamin C: 28 mg	Fat: 2 g

LUNCH OR DINNER DISHES AND SIDES

BELINDA'S BAKED BEANS

1 30-oz can pork and beans (discard pork)	1/8 tsp ground cloves
1/4 cup catsup	1/8 tsp cinnamon
1 medium onion, chopped	1/8 tsp black pepper
1 red pepper, chopped	1/2 tsp salt (optional)
2 tbsp brown sugar	1 tsp sweet pickle juice (optional)
1 tsp dry mustard	

Combine all ingredients in 1-quart baking dish. Bake at 300°F for 30 minutes. Serves 8.

Nutrients per serving

Calories: 157	Carbohydrates: 31 g	Protein: 6 g
Saturated fat: 0	Monounsaturated fat: 0	Cholesterol: 0
Fiber: 6 g	Fat: 1 g	

Comment: Belinda, a research dietitian with our group, recommends this very easy phytochemical-rich main dish.

GLAZED SNOW PEAS AND CARROTS

4 tsp cornstarch
1 16-oz can fat-free, reduced-sodium chicken broth, divided
1 tsp lemon juice

4 medium carrots (about 2 cups), sliced diagonally
1 medium red onion (about ½ cup), coarsely chopped
8 oz (about 2 cups) snow peas

In cup, stir together cornstarch, ½ cup chicken broth, and lemon juice until smooth; set aside. In 10-inch skillet over high heat, heat remaining broth to boiling. Add carrots and onion; cook until carrots are tender-crisp, stirring occasionally. Add snow peas; cook 2 minutes. Reduce heat to medium. Stir cornstarch mixture into skillet. Cook until mixture boils and thickens, stirring constantly. Serves 5.

Nutrients per serving

Calories: 79	Carbohydrates: 16 g	Protein: 4 g
Saturated fat: 0	Monounsaturated fat: 0	Cholesterol: 0
Fiber: 4 g	Beta-carotene: 2 mg	Vitamin C: 37 mg
Fat: 0		

VEGETABLE MEDLEY

1 16-oz can fat-free, chicken broth
1 cup broccoli florets
1 cup cauliflower florets

1 medium carrot (about ½ cup), sliced
1 celery stalk (about ½ cup), sliced

In 3-quart saucepan over high heat, heat broth and vegetables to boiling. Reduce heat to low. Cover; cook 5 minutes or until vegetables are tender-crisp. Drain and serve. Serves 6.

Nutrients per serving

Calories: 29	Carbohydrates: 5 g	Protein: 3 g
Saturated fat: 0	Monounsaturated fat: 0	Cholesterol: 0
Fiber: 2 g	Vitamin C: 41 mg	Fat: 0

SUMMER MIXED GREENS

8 cups packed mixed greens, coarsely chopped (spinach, kale, mustard, turnip, etc.)	1 clove garlic, minced
	1 tbsp cider vinegar
	1/2 tsp red pepper flakes
2 tsp olive oil	1/2 tsp salt
1/2 cup onion, finely chopped	2 cups water
1/2 cup celery, finely chopped	

Clean and wash greens; drain thoroughly. Heat oil in a slow cooker over medium heat. Add onions, celery, and garlic and cook for 5 minutes, stirring occasionally. Stir in the greens; cover and cook for 10 minutes until greens are wilted, stirring occasionally. Add vinegar, pepper flakes, and salt; cover and cook for 5 minutes. Add 2 cups water, cover, and simmer for 2 hours, adding more water if necessary. Serve with additional vinegar if desired. Serves 6.

Nutrients per serving

Calories: 55	Carbohydrates: 9 g	Protein: 2 g
Saturated fat: 0	Monounsaturated fat: 0	Cholesterol: 0
Fiber: 3	Vitamin C: 27 mg	Fat: 2 g

MAIN DISHES: LUNCH OR DINNER

RED PEPPER PIZZA

1 refrigerated pizza crust	2 tbsp minced fresh basil
5 sweet red peppers, thinly sliced	Crushed pepper flakes (optional)
3 cloves garlic, minced	

On a pizza tin, roll out dough as directed on package. In a large, nonstick skillet over medium heat, sauté the peppers and garlic, stirring often, for 7 to 10 minutes. Remove from heat and stir in basil and pepper flakes. Spread crust with pepper mixture. Bake at 450° to 500°F for 15 minutes or until crust is brown or crispy. (You may need to modify baking time according to instructions on pizza crust package.) Serves 4.

Nutrients per serving

Calories: 246	Carbohydrates: 47 g	Protein: 8 g
Saturated fat: 0	Monounsaturated fat: 0	Cholesterol: 0
Fiber: 4 g	Beta-carotene: 7 mg	Vitamin C: 427 mg
Fat: 21 g		

SOY GOOD PIZZA

1 cup textured soy protein hydrated with 1 cup boiling water	2 cloves garlic, minced
	1 tsp black pepper
	1 bay leaf
1 28-oz can Italian-style tomato puree	1 refrigerated pizza crust
2 tsp finely chopped hot chili peppers	

Hydrate soy protein and set aside. Combine all ingredients except pizza dough into 3-quart saucepan, cover, and bring to a boil. Uncover, lower the heat, and simmer for 30 minutes, stirring occasionally. On a pizza tin, roll out dough as directed on package. Spoon the sauce over the pizza dough. Bake at 450° to 500°F for 15 minutes or until crust is brown or crispy. (You may need to modify baking time according to instructions on pizza crust package.) Serves 8.

Nutrients per serving

Calories: 255	Carbohydrates: 45 g	Protein: 15 g
Saturated fat: 0	Monounsaturated fat: 0	Cholesterol: 0
Fiber: 4 g	Soy protein: 6 g	Vitamin C: 36 mg
Fat: 2 g		

Comment: Your friends will think this is made from hamburger and enjoy the spicy flavor.

RED PEPPER SPAGHETTI

1 medium onion, chopped
(½ cup)
1 red pepper, without seeds,
chopped
1 carton (10.25-oz) extra-firm
tofu, cut into ½-inch cubes

½ cup black olives, sliced and
pitted
1 15.5-oz jar spaghetti sauce
6 cups cooked spaghetti

Sauté onion and pepper in skillet sprayed with canola nonstick cooking spray. Add tofu, olives, and spaghetti sauce. Bring to boil, mix, and let simmer for 10 minutes. Serve over hot spaghetti. Serves 6.

Comment: Son-in-law Tom has an Italian mother and grew up with good Italian food. This spaghetti sauce is one of his favorites, which he often prepares for the family.

Nutrients per serving

Calories: 315
Saturated fat: 2 g
Fiber: 5 g
Fat: 8 g

Carbohydrates: 49 g
Monounsaturated fat: 3 g
Soy protein: 6 g

Protein: 13 g
Cholesterol: 0
Vitamin C: 69 mg

GINGERED BROCCOLI WITH PASTA

1 bunch broccoli (1½ lb)
1½ cups chicken broth, divided
2 tbsp olive oil
1 tbsp minced fresh ginger
1 tsp minced garlic
⅛ tsp crushed red pepper

¼ tsp salt
1 lb fusilli, rotelle, or radiatore
pasta, cooked according to
package directions
Parmesan cheese (optional)

Cut broccoli from stems into small florets. Peel and slice stems. Process sliced stems and ½ cup chicken broth until very fine. Heat olive oil in large skillet over medium-high heat. Add ginger, garlic, and red pepper; cook 15 seconds. Stir in pureed broccoli mixture, florets, remaining 1 cup chicken broth, and salt. Boil, stirring occasionally, just until broccoli is tender, 5 to 8 minutes. Toss with pasta. Makes 6 servings. Sprinkle with Parmesan cheese, as desired.

Nutrients per serving

Calories: 277	Carbohydrates: 38 g	Protein: 11 g
Saturated fat: 1 g	Monounsaturated fat: 4 g	Cholesterol: 1 mg
Fiber: 5 g	Vitamin C: 119 mg	Fat: 9 g

MARINARA SAUCE

Olive oil- or canola oil-flavored cooking spray
1 cup sweet red pepper, chopped
1 medium onion, chopped (1/2 cup)
2 tbsp chopped fresh parsley (optional)
1 clove garlic, minced
1 29-oz can tomato sauce
1 14 1/2-oz can Italian-stewed tomatoes, chopped, undrained

1 tsp sugar
1/2 tsp dried oregano leaves
1/2 tsp dried basil leaves
1/2 tsp dried thyme leaves
1/4 tsp salt
1/4 tsp black pepper, ground
8 scoops (4 oz) soy nutritious food ingredient*
Pasta to serve

Coat a small saucepan with cooking spray. Combine pepper, onion, parsley, and garlic in saucepan; spray vegetables with cooking spray. Cook with medium heat until onion is tender, stirring frequently. Stir in next 8 ingredients; bring to a boil. Reduce heat to low, cover, and simmer 20 minutes. Remove from heat; stir in soy food ingredient. Serve over the pasta of your choice. Serves 4.

Nutrients per serving

Calories: 299	Carbohydrates: 59 g	Protein: 11 g
Saturated fat: 0	Monounsaturated fat: 1 g	Cholesterol: 0
Fiber: 8 g	Soy protein: 10 g	Beta-carotene: 2 mg
Vitamin C: 99 mg	Fat: 2 g	

*Available from Nutritious Foods, Inc., 4600 Chippewa, No. 281, St. Louis, MO 63116; tel. 1-800-445-3350.

VEGETARIAN LASAGNA

9 lasagna noodles
1 tbsp olive or canola oil
1 medium onion, chopped
4 large mushrooms (8 oz), sliced
1 clove garlic, minced
1 carton (10.25-oz) soft tofu, cut into 1/2-inch cubes
1/4 cup Parmesan cheese, grated
2 tsp fresh parsley, chopped

1/2 tsp salt
1/4 tsp black pepper
1/4 tsp dried oregano
10 oz frozen chopped broccoli, thawed and squeezed of excess liquid
3 cups spaghetti sauce
1/4 cup part-skim mozzarella cheese, grated

Cook lasagna noodles; set aside. Heat oil in skillet for 1 minute over medium heat. Sauté onions, mushrooms, and garlic until onions are tender. In a bowl, mix together tofu, Parmesan cheese, parsley, salt, pepper, and oregano. Mix onion mixture, tofu mixture, and broccoli. Spray an 8 × 11-inch baking dish with canola nonstick spray. Spread 1/2 cup tomato sauce in bottom of baking dish. Place 3 noodles on top of sauce. Spread half of broccoli-onion-tofu mixture on noodles. Spoon 1/2 cup sauce over broccoli mixture; place 3 noodles on top. Spread with remaining broccoli mixture; top with 1/2 cup sauce. Top with remaining noodles and sauce; sprinkle with mozzarella cheese. Cover with foil. Bake at 350°F for 40 minutes in preheated oven. Remove foil, bake another 10 minutes, and serve. Serves 8.

Nutrients per serving

Calories: 247	Carbohydrates: 35 g	Protein: 12 g
Saturated fat: 1 g	Monounsaturated fat: 2 g	Cholesterol: 20 mg
Fiber: 5 g	Soy protein: 3 g	Vitamin C: 45 mg
Fat: 6 g		

Comment: Tofu makes an excellent cheese substitute in this recipe.

Easy Vegetable Primavera

1 16-oz can low-sodium chicken broth, divided	2 tbsp cornstarch
1/2 tsp minced garlic	10 1/4 oz firm tofu cut into 1/2-inch cubes
2 cups broccoli florets	4 cups hot spaghetti (about 8 oz, dry)
1 cup carrots, sliced diagonally	
1/2 cup red pepper strips	1 tbsp grated Parmesan cheese (optional)
1 small onion, chopped	

In 2-quart saucepan over high heat, heat 1 cup chicken broth and garlic to boiling. Stir in broccoli, carrots, pepper, and onion. Reduce heat to medium. Cover; cook 5 minutes until vegetables are tender-crisp. In cup, stir together cornstarch and remaining chicken broth until smooth; stir into vegetable mixture. Cook until mixture boils and thickens, stirring constantly. Gently stir in tofu; heat through. Serve over spaghetti. Sprinkle with cheese. Serves 5.

Nutrients per serving

Calories: 264	Carbohydrates: 43 g	Protein: 15 g
Saturated fat: 1 g	Monounsaturated fat: 1 g	Cholesterol: 0
Fiber: 4 g	Soy protein: 7 g	Vitamin C: 56 mg
Fat: 4 g		

DOWN HOME CHILI

1   cup textured soy protein,
    mixed with 1 cup boiling
    water, set aside
2   16-oz cans whole tomatoes,
    crushed
1   3-oz can tomato paste
1   large onion, chopped
1   red pepper, chopped
1   jalepeño pepper, minced

2   tbsp chili powder
1   to 2 tsp cumin powder
2   tsp garlic powder
1   tsp oregano
¼   tsp allspice
1   15½-oz can kidney or pinto
    beans
1   15-oz can black beans

Add first 11 ingredients to a large saucepan and simmer, covered, for 1 hour. Add beans and simmer for 30 to 60 minutes longer. Serve in bowls. Serves 6.

Comment: For variety, serve over hot rice or spaghetti. Make ahead of time because this chili is better when reheated the next day.

Nutrients per serving

Calories: 272
Saturated fat: 0
Fiber: 13 g
Fat: 2 g

Carbohydrates: 46 g
Monounsaturated fat: 0
Soy protein: 9 g

Protein: 22 g
Cholesterol: 0
Vitamin C: 91 mg

VEGETARIAN TACOS

1 cup textured soy protein
1 cup boiling water
1 package (4 oz) taco
   seasoning
12 oz vegetarian refried beans
12 taco shells, baked
1 cup (4 oz) fat-free cheddar
   cheese

1 medium tomato, chopped
   (½ cup)
1 medium onion, chopped
   (½ cup)
½ cup lettuce, shredded
Taco sauce, as desired

Place soy protein in mixing bowl and add boiling water; mix in taco seasoning. Heat taco mixture, beans, and taco shells. Spread taco mixture, beans, cheese, tomatoes, onions, and lettuce in taco shell. Add taco sauce, as desired. Serves 6.

Nutrients per serving

Calories: 290
Saturated fat: 1 g
Fiber: 9 g

Carbohydrates: 37 g
Monounsaturated fat: 3 g
Soy protein: 9 g

Protein: 23 g
Cholesterol: 0
Fat: 7 g

SESAME TOFU STIR-FRY

1 carton (10.25-oz) extra-firm
   tofu, cut into ½-inch cubes
2 tbsp reduced-sodium soy
   sauce
1 tsp hot sesame oil
1 tbsp canola oil
1 medium onion, chopped
   (½ cup)

1 garlic clove, diced
2 medium-sweet red peppers,
   cut in thin strips
1 cup carrots, sliced
2 cups broccoli, chopped
4 cups cooked rice

Mix soy sauce and sesame oil in small baking dish; add tofu and coat with sauce. Refrigerate for 30 to 60 minutes. Heat wok or skillet to medium hot, add canola oil, and heat for 1 minute. Add onion and garlic and sauté until onion is tender. Add peppers, carrots, and broccoli, and cook until crispy-tender. Add tofu and sauce; stir gently. Cover and let simmer for 10 minutes. Serves 4.

Nutrients per serving

Calories: 399	Carbohydrates: 62 g	Protein: 17 g
Saturated fat: 1 g	Monounsaturated fat: 3 g	Cholesterol: 0
Fiber: 5 g	Soy protein: 9 g	Beta-carotene: 4 mg
Vitamin C: 218 mg	Fat: 10 g	

VEGETABLE TOFU STIR-FRY

1 tbsp canola oil	¼ cup stir-fry sauce
1 carton (10.25-oz) extra-firm tofu, cut into ½-inch cubes	4 cups cooked rice
1 package (16-oz) frozen mixed vegetables	

Heat oil in large skillet or wok until hot. Add tofu and stir-fry for 3 minutes. Add frozen vegetables and sauce and stir-fry for 6 to 8 minutes until vegetable colors intensify. Serve immediately over rice. Serves 4.

Nutrients per serving

Calories: 396	Carbohydrates: 63 g	Protein: 18 g	Fat: 8 g
Saturated fat: 0	Monounsaturated fat: 2 g	Cholesterol: 0	
Fiber: 4 g	Soy protein: 9 g	Beta-carotene: 8 mg	

Comment: This quick and easy recipe is a favorite at our house. I often fix it when Gay is gone and omit the rice; I can eat the whole thing and not exceed my calorie limit. The tofu can be stored for months in the refrigerator, and the vegetables are frozen. Keep the ingredients on hand for a fast meal.

SWEET AND SOUR TOFU

Sauce

¼ cup pineapple juice	¼ cup catsup
4 tbsp brown sugar	1 tbsp cornstarch
5 tbsp sugar	
2 tbsp reduced-sodium soy sauce	

Combine all ingredients, mix thoroughly, and set aside.

1 tbsp canola oil	1 large green pepper, in long, thin slices
1 medium onion, thinly sliced	
2 medium carrots, sliced diagonally	2 medium zucchini, cut in rounds
1 large red pepper, in long, thin slices	1 10¼-oz carton firm tofu
	1 4-oz can pineapple chunks

In a large wok or skillet, heat oil and add onions; sauté for several minutes until translucent. Add carrots and peppers; sauté for a few minutes; add zucchini. Turn down heat, cover, and simmer, stirring once or twice, until vegetables are tender-crisp. Add tofu, pineapple, and sauce and bring to a boil. Simmer, stirring gently, for 3 to 4 minutes. Serve over rice or noodles. Serves 4.

Nutrients per serving

Calories: 316	Carbohydrates: 55 g	Protein: 12 g
Saturated fat: 1 g	Monounsaturated fat: 2 g	Cholesterol: 0
Fiber: 4 g	Soy protein: 9 g	Vitamin C: 118 mg
Fat: 6 g		

Comment: This colorful dish is rich in antioxidants and easy to prepare.

SLOPPY JOE SURPRISE

1 cup textured soy protein	1 tbsp Worcestershire sauce
7/8 cup boiling water	2 tbsp brown sugar
2 tbsp canola oil	1/2 tsp salt
1 cup chopped onions	Freshly ground pepper to
1 large green pepper, coarsely	taste
chopped	Tabasco sauce to taste
2 cups tomato sauce	(optional)
1 to 1 1/2 tbsp chili powder	4 hamburger rolls

Pour the boiling water over the textured soy protein and set aside. Heat oil in large skillet and add onions and pepper; sauté until they are tender. Stir in the textured soy protein and other ingredients. Cover and simmer for 20 minutes. Serves 4.

Nutrients per serving

Calories: 503	Carbohydrates: 73 g	Protein: 24 g
Saturated fat: 2 g	Monounsaturated fat: 8 g	Cholesterol: 0
Fiber: 7 g	Soy protein: 14 g	Vitamin C: 44 mg
Fat: 15 g		

Comment: Our New Jersey visitor who was uncertain about the identity of tofu was pleased with these sloppy joes.

TOFU SWEET POTATO BAKE

1 10 1/4-oz carton silken (low-	1/4 tsp salt
fat) tofu	1 tsp cinnamon
1 15-oz can sweet potatoes	1/8 tsp ginger
2 tbsp brown sugar	

Add all ingredients to a blender and blend until smooth. Pour into casserole dish and bake for 20 minutes at 350°F in preheated oven. Serves 6.

Nutrients per serving

Calories: 112	Carbohydrates: 21 g	Protein: 5 g
Saturated fat: 0	Monounsaturated fat: 0	Cholesterol: 0
Fiber: 2 g	Soy protein: 4 g	Fat: 1 g

SNACKS AND RECIPES FOR ANY MEAL

BLACK BEAN DIP

1 15-oz can black beans, drained	1/3 cup mild picante sauce
1 tsp canola oil	1/2 tsp ground cumin
1 medium onion, chopped	1/2 tsp chili powder
2 garlic cloves, minced	1/4 cup (1 oz) reduced-fat Monterey Jack cheese, shredded
1/2 cup fresh or canned tomatoes, chopped	1 tbsp lime juice

Place beans in bowl, partially mash until chunky, and set aside.

Spray nonstick medium skillet with canola nonstick spray. Heat oil over medium heat and add onion and garlic. Sauté for about 4 minutes or until tender. Add beans, tomatoes, and next three ingredients. Cook 5 minutes or until thickened, stirring constantly. Remove from heat, add cheese and lime juice, and stir until cheese is melted. Serve warm or at room temperature with fat-free corn chips. Makes 1⅔ cups or about 24 1-tbsp servings.

Nutrients per serving

Calories: 30	Carbohydrates: 5 g	Protein: 2 g
Saturated fat: 0	Monounsaturated fat: 0	Cholesterol: 0
Fiber: 1 g	Fat: 0	

BEVERAGES, DESSERTS, OR SNACKS

TUTTI-FRUITTI

1 cup skim milk
½ banana
½ cup fresh or frozen
   unsweetened strawberries (do
   not thaw)

2 scoops (2 oz) strawberry
   high soy protein nutritious
   beverage powder*
1 10-oz bottle cherry-flavored
   sparkling water, chilled

Combine first 4 ingredients in container of electric blender; top with cover, and process until smooth. Divide mixture into 2 12-oz glasses. Stir 5 ounces water into each glass. Serves 2.

Nutrients per serving

Calories: 236   Carbohydrates: 43 g   Protein: 14 g
Saturated fat: 0   Monounsaturated fat: 0   Cholesterol: 2 mg
Fiber: 1 g   Soy protein: 10 g   Fat: 1 g

*Available from Nutritious Foods, Inc., 4600 Chippewa, No 281, St. Louis, MO 63116; tel. 1-800-445-3350.

STRAWBERRY-BANANA FROSTY

3 cups plain or vanilla soy milk
   (beverage)

1 ripe banana
1 cup strawberries

Blend in blender until smooth. Serves 4.

Nutrients per serving

Calories: 140   Carbohydrates: 8 g   Protein: 20 g
Saturated fat: 0   Monounsaturated fat: 1 g   Cholesterol: 0
Fiber: 1 g   Soy protein: 8 g   Vitamin C: 24 mg
Fat: 3 g

Comment: This beverage also can make a quick, low-calorie breakfast.

Tangy Vegetable Juice

2 12-oz cans vegetable juice
1 tsp prepared horseradish
1 tsp Worcestershire sauce

$\frac{1}{2}$ tsp hot pepper sauce
4 lemon slices

In pitcher combine first 4 ingredients and stir. Serve over ice cubes with lemon slices. Serves 4.

Nutrients per serving

Calories: 42	Carbohydrates: 10 g	Protein: 1 g
Saturated fat: 0	Monounsaturated fat: 0	Cholesterol: 0
Fiber: 2	Vitamin C: 43 mg	Fat: 0

DESSERTS

Soy-Good Chocolate Pudding

$\frac{1}{3}$ cup honey
$\frac{1}{4}$ cup cocoa powder
$1\frac{1}{2}$ tsp vanilla

1 $10\frac{1}{4}$-oz package low-fat, silken tofu, drained

Heat honey for 90 seconds in microwave. Pour over cocoa powder; add vanilla. Stir until smooth. Blend tofu until soft. Add chocolate mixture and continue blending for 1 minute. Chill for at least 1 hour. Serves 5.

Nutrients per serving

Calories: 112	Carbohydrates: 21 g	Protein: 5 g
Saturated fat: 0	Monounsaturated fat: 0	Cholesterol: 0
Fiber: 0	Soy protein: 5 g	Fat: 1 g

Comment: Teresa served this at one of our staff meetings and won rave reviews; then she told us it was made with soy. Her teenage daughter won't let this pudding reside in the refrigerator for very long.

CITRUS SURPRISE

2 oranges, peeled and sectioned
1 grapefruit, peeled and sectioned
1 kiwi, peeled and sliced

1 tbsp sugar-free instant vanilla pudding
½ cup nonfat yogurt
¼ cup orange juice

Prepare fruit and place in 1-quart bowl. Whisk pudding in small amount of yogurt to disperse. Add yogurt and pudding to juice and mix until smooth. Add fruit and mix. Cover and refrigerate 30 minutes or until chilled. Serves 4.

Nutrients per serving

Calories: 104
Saturated fat: 0
Fiber: 6 g

Carbohydrates: 24 g
Monounsaturated fat: 0
Vitamin C: 104 mg

Protein 3 g
Cholesterol: 0
Fat: 0

Comment: It doesn't get much simpler than this. This is one of my favorite quick and easy desserts.

PUMPKIN PIE

Shell

2 cups rolled oats
½ cup whole-wheat flour
1 tsp cinnamon (to taste)
½ tsp vanilla extract

2 tbsp canola oil
1 tbsp honey
3 tbsp water

Combine all ingredients and mix well; press into bottom of 9- to 10-inch pie pan. Mix will be crumbly.

Filling

 2 15-oz cans pumpkin
 1 10.5-oz carton soft tofu
 2 tsp sweetener
 ½ tsp salt

 ½ tsp ginger
 ½ tsp ground cloves
 1 tbsp vanilla extract

Combine all filling ingredients with an electric mixer or food processor. Pour mixture into pie shell. Bake for 1 hour at 350°F in a preheated oven. Serves 6.

Nutrients per serving

Calories: 231   Carbohydrates: 34 g   Protein: 9 g   Fat: 7 g
Saturated fat: 1 g   Monounsaturated fat: 4 g   Cholesterol: 0
Fiber: 7 g   Soy protein: 4 g

10

WALK FOR THE HEALTH OF IT: REDUCE RISKS OF DEBILITATING DISEASE

- Forget "No pain, no gain."
- Remember "Use it or lose it."

More than 450 years ago, in the first book devoted totally to exercise, Cristobol Mendez wrote: "The best and most beneficial exercise is walking."[1] Dr. Kenneth Cooper, the father of "aerobics" and long-time advocate of running, recently said: "I think people should walk more and run less."[1] Walking and other aerobic exercises promote health and reduce risk for many diseases of aging. Recent studies show that older individuals who have exercised regularly throughout their adult life have physical endurances, muscle strength, and flexibilities that exceed those of much younger people who have "couch potato" lifestyles.[2] Scientists have been awestruck by the physical capabilities of some octogenerians who have maintained active lifestyles in recent years. As we will share with you in this chapter, walking a moderate amount (at least twelve miles per week) enhances your health and longevity, while brisk walking (five miles per hour) for at least twenty miles per week increases health, longevity, and physical fitness. For weight loss and long-term weight maintenance, walking at least one hour per day (about thirty to thirty-five miles per week) is necessary for most people.

HEALTH BENEFITS OF EXERCISE

Let's review some of the health benefits of regular aerobic exercise before talking about the best forms of exercise and the amount you need to do. Regular aerobic exercise:

- reduces the risk for heart attack or stroke;
- decreases the risk for developing cancer, especially those of the colon, breast, prostate, and lung;
- lowers the risk for adult-onset diabetes;
- drops blood pressure;
- assists in weight maintenance;
- protects from osteoporosis;
- contributes to peaceful living;
- prolongs life and enhances the quality of life.*

Regular aerobic exercise decreases risk for developing these health problems: heart attack and strokes; a wide variety of cancers but, especially, colon, breast, prostate, and lung cancers; adult-onset diabetes (noninsulin-dependent diabetes mellitus); high blood pressure; obesity; and osteoporosis. In addition, regular exercise assists in stress management and peaceful living. The bottom line, however, is that exercise prolongs life and enhances its quality. All of these benefits represent a pretty good return on an investment of thirty minutes per day.[3,4]

* From Blair et al.[3] and other sources.

EXERCISE AND FREE RADICALS

When we exercise, the muscles require large amounts of oxygen; this accounts for the heavy breathing or panting I sometimes do when I push myself too hard on a stair machine or a rowing machine. As muscles suck up all this oxygen, they also generate free radicals. Very vigorous aerobic exercise, such as running as hard and as fast as you can, delivers enormous quantities of oxygen to the muscles and exposes them to damage by the large numbers of free radicals being formed. Often there are not adequate amounts of antioxidants in muscle to protect from free radical damage. This free radical damage contributes to the soreness and swelling of muscles after unusually heavy exercise. Walking and less strenuous exercise do not overtax the capacity of muscles to neutralize free radicals with antioxidants and thus are less likely to result in muscle damage.

Free radicals and antioxidants occupy a prominent place in thinking about the protective benefits of regular exercise. Previously it was felt that exercise increased blood supply to the heart and thus decreased risk for heart attack. Now experts suspect that exercise is diverting oxygen and free radicals to the muscles so they do not damage blood vessels. Likewise, in the cancer area previous thinking suggested that exercise decreased body weight and thus decreased risk for cancer. Now experts propose that exercise directs oxygen and free radicals into exercising muscles, thereby protecting more vulnerable tissues from damage from these reckless particles.

EXERCISE AND THE HEART

Regular exercise offers many bonuses to the heart and circulatory system. Exercise fine-tunes the fat particles in the blood by decreasing the "bad guy" LDL particles and increasing the "good guy" HDL particles. Exercise also lowers the triglycerides that can contribute to hardening of the arteries. Furthermore, exercise decreases blood clotting and platelet stickiness, thereby lessening chances of blood clot formation in blood vessels in the heart or brain.[4] As discussed in Chapter 3, blood clots or thromboses are the major causes of heart attacks or strokes.

Through a program of aerobic exercise the heart grows stronger with increased blood supply and is less vulnerable to a reduction in blood flow if a blood vessel becomes clogged. Exercise also slows down the heart rate and lowers the blood pressure, thus decreasing the work of the heart. In addition, regular exercise lowers blood insulin levels; recent research indicates that high blood insulin levels lead to high blood pressure, high blood triglyceride levels, and increased risk for heart attack.[4]

EXERCISE AND CANCER

Regular exercise decreases risk from death from all causes, including cancer.[5-8] Blair and colleagues[3] reviewed the research relating physical activity to various types of cancers and found substantial evidence that exercise reduces risk for all forms of cancer. They rated the evidence as: 0 (inconclusive); + (some evidence); ++ (good evidence); and +++ (excellent evidence). For example, the relationship between exercise and decreased heart attack rates was rated +++. For cancers they provide the following ratings: all cause, +; colon, ++; rectum, 0; breast, +; prostate, +; and lung, +. Thus regular exercise seems to reduce risk for all types of cancer and seems to have the greatest protective effect against colon, breast, prostate, and lung cancers.

EXERCISE AND DIABETES

The adult-onset type of diabetes is very common in the United States and is increasing dramatically in many emerging countries, such as Mexico. Obesity, high fat intake, and low fiber intake appear to play major roles in development of diabetes.[4] Resistance of skeletal muscle to the action of insulin has a major role in development of adult-type diabetes. High levels of physical activity have been linked to protection from diabetes for many years, but convincing evidence has emerged only recently. A recent study of alumni of the University of Pennsylvania[9] demonstrated that the rates of development of diabetes were inversely related to the level of physical activity for these men. The prevalence rate decreased about 6 percent for every five miles walked per week. Men who still participated in vigorous sports such as swimming or tennis developed diabetes at less than half the rate for sedentary men.

EXERCISE AND BLOOD PRESSURE

Regular aerobic exercise significantly decreases blood pressure. The reductions in systolic blood pressure (the upper number) are approximately 4 to 5 millimeters of mercury (mm Hg) or 3 percent below initial levels, while the decreases in diastolic blood pressure (the lower number) are approximately 2 to 3 mm Hg or 2 percent.[4] Even these modest reductions in blood pressure can reduce estimated risk for heart attack by 5 to 10 percent. Of course, remaining slender, eating high-fiber foods, and obtaining generous amounts of potassium and magnesium also lower blood pressure.[4]

EXERCISE AND WEIGHT CONTROL

Some slender people are quite active, while some obese people are quite sedentary. Serious obesity severely limits physical activity. Regular exercise is an essential part of successful weight loss and weight maintenance.[10, 11] While these general statements seem reasonable, much more research is required to link decreased physical activity to increased body weight.[3, 11] Whether a person is slender or overweight, regular exercise improves his or her health and longevity.[11] Recent research indicates that an exercise program involving low- to moderate-intensity exercise must be performed almost daily for at least an hour per session to successfully promote weight loss and weight maintenance.[11]

HOW MUCH EXERCISE SHOULD I DO?

You probably are wondering how many miles you need to log each week to get these health benefits. The more you walk, the more health benefits you receive, up to a total of thirty-five miles per week.[7] Figure 10.1 illustrates the longevity benefits of regular physical activity. The lowest level of fitness (rated a 1) represents walking fewer than five miles per week. The midrange (rated 2 to 3) represents walking approximately five to twenty miles per week, while the high range (rated 4 to 5) represents walking approximately twenty to thirty-five miles per week. Several studies[5–8] indicate that the major health advantage is achieved with exercise levels equivalent to walking about twelve to fourteen miles per week and that increases to about thirty-five miles per week are associated with only small increases in health benefits. Figure 10.2 illustrates health advantages achieved by walking or running varying distances per week. Of great

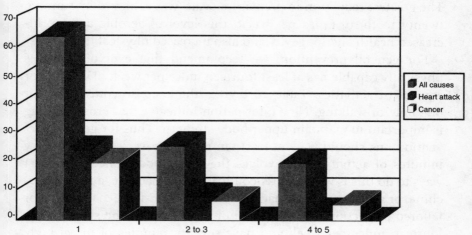

FIGURE 10.1   *Rates of Death in Men Adjusted for Age Based on Level of Physical Fitness.*

Rates are expressed as deaths per 10,000 person-years of follow-up. Data from Cooper Clinic with level of fitness rated from 1 (low) to 5 (high).[8]

importance, a 55 percent reduction in premature death rates was achieved with walks of two to three miles on three or four days per week, with a total distance covered of only six to ten miles per week.

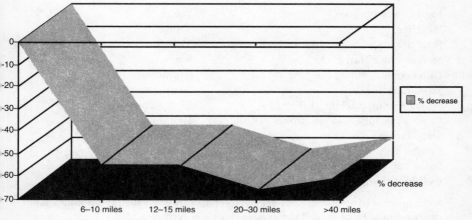

FIGURE 10.2   *Reduction in Premature Deaths Related to Miles Walked or Run per Week*

The greatest reduction in premature death was achieved by running twenty to thirty miles per week; this level of aerobic activity increased health and longevity and also increased physical fitness.

For general prevention, we recommend that everyone who is physically capable has at least fourteen miles per week of walking or equivalent activities. Table 10.1 gives the exercise equivalents for one mile of walking. New information indicates that cross-training is important to maintain upper-body strength. Thus for general prevention one should walk at least ten miles per week and have forty minutes of activity that involves the upper body; one of the best ways to do this is with a cross-country skiing machine, a rowing machine, or a sitting rowing machine (such as an E-force machine). For tailored protection or for reversal of heart disease one should walk fourteen miles per week and have seventy minutes of upper-body exercise. During weight loss and weight maintenance, the most successful people walk at least twenty-one miles per week and do seventy minutes of upper-body exercise per week.[10]

TABLE 10.1   DIFFERENT FORMS OF EXERCISE THAT ARE EQUIVALENT TO WALKING ONE MILE

ACTIVITY	TIME OR DISTANCE EQUIVALENT TO WALKING ONE MILE*
Jogging or running	1 mile
Bicycling	3 miles
Stair climbing	25 flights
Stair machine (fast pace)	8 minutes
Cross-country skiing machine	8 minutes
Swimming	10 minutes
Sitting rowing machine (E-Force)	10 minutes
Rowing machine (twenty strokes per minute)	10 minutes
Stationary bicycle	12 minutes
Aerobic dancing	12 minutes
Basketball (noncompetitive)	12 minutes
Golf (not riding a cart)	20 minutes

* The amount of aerobic activity acheived (or activity equivalent to walking 1 mile) depends on the intensity of the exercise for most activities.

WHAT TYPE OF EXERCISE SHOULD I DO?

Good forms of aerobic activity are walking, jogging, cycling (outdoors or with an Exercycle), swimming, cross-country skiing (most use a machine), or rowing. For most people we recommend walking two to three miles per day and getting ten to twenty minutes of upper-body exercise per day. For general prevention we recommend walking two miles daily for five days per week (walking at least ten miles weekly) and doing ten minutes of upper-body exercise four days weekly. For upper-body exercise we recommend a rowing machine, a sitting rowing machine (such as a Cardioglide or E-Force machine), a cross-country skiing machine (such as a Nordic Track), or swimming.

HOW SHOULD I START
MY EXERCISE PROGRAM?

Walking is your best exercise. Probably you already are walking some—to your car, in the supermarket, and at work. Estimate how many minutes you walk per day; chances are you walk a mile in twenty to twenty-five minutes. If you currently are walking about ten minutes per day (let's say that is one-half mile), could you increase that by five minutes? In the first week, try to walk 50 percent more than you currently are doing. Remember that the minimum amount of walking that *may* provide health benefits is one mile per day, six days per week (see Figure 10.2). However, most research suggests that you need to walk twelve miles per week to achieve a definite health advantage. If your physical condition permits, try to gradually increase your walking to two miles per day, six days per week.

Before starting your walking program you need to get some good running shoes. Yes, running shoes. Your old tennis shoes, work shoes, or dress shoes just won't be friendly to your feet. Go to a store that sells running shoes and ask the manager to recommend shoes that support your own walking style best. Owners or managers of stores selling good running shoes can recommend your best choices. Casey Meyers provides detailed advice about selecting appropriate walking shoes.[1]

You need to find ways to increase your physical activity in your everyday life. Park at the extreme corner of the parking lot at work, at the restaurant, and at the shopping mall. Walk the stairs when you get a chance. Four flights of stairs three times daily represents the equivalent of one-half mile and takes much less than ten minutes. Program in extra walking at the supermarket by going down extra aisles rather than going right to the familiar aisles that have your requirements. Try to find errands that require extra walking; hand-deliver the letter rather than putting it in the office mail.

You'll thank us after you have established your schedule of walking one to three miles per day. You will sleep better, have more energy, and protect your health and longevity. Soon you will want to go for physical fitness as well as for health and longevity. Remember, though, that "no pain, no gain" is not our motto. Gradually increase your exercise so you do not have sore muscles and do not burn out. This is a life-long venture you're starting, so go slow and easy.

TO SUM UP

- Regular exercise improves health, reduces risk for diseases, and increases longevity.
- Moderate levels of aerobic exercise improve health *and* physical fitness.

WHAT YOU CAN DO

- Increase your walking time by 50 percent this week.
- Find ways to work more walking into your daily schedule.

JIM'S DIARY

Recently my doctor sent me to take a stress test. While I felt that my lower chest distress was related to my hiatal hernia, he wanted to be sure I wasn't having heart pain. The test provided good news and bad news. First, the good news: At age fifty-nine and with a history of a high blood cholesterol, my stress test was entirely negative. The heart tracing (EKG) and echo machine showed nothing that suggested heart disease. My cardiology friend who did the test says he feels certain that I do not have any meaningful blockage in the blood vessels to my heart. I was pleased and reassured by this test. So, what is the bad news? During the stress test my heart rate and blood pressure went up to high levels very quickly. This means that my physical conditioning is not very good. Although I walk more than three miles a day and log about twenty-five miles per week, I do not do aerobic walking on a regular basis. This test told me that I need to increase my aerobic conditioning. I also need to do something to maintain my upper-body conditioning. As a result, I purchased an E-force sitting rowing machine and started at the beginning level (see Table 8.1) by doing five to seven minutes daily. After a few weeks my repetitions per minute had doubled without my heart racing. Already my cardiovascular fitness has improved. And I still walk at least twenty-five miles per week.

11

HEALTHY SHOPPING, COOKING, AND EATING OUT

While practicing what is recommended in *Dr. Anderson's Antioxidant, Antiaging Health Program,* it is okay to enjoy all aspects of life, including shopping, cooking, and eating.

SHOPPING MADE EASY

Shopping at modern-day supermarkets often seems like an overwhelming task because we are faced with such an overwhelming plethora of choices. The typical supermarket has more than twenty-six thousand foods on its shelves, and that's not counting tens of thousands of nonfood items such as lightbulbs, paper towels, laundry detergent, and other cleaning supplies. Here's a suggestion: Since *Dr. Anderson's Antioxidant Antiaging Health Program* emphasizes antioxidant- and phytochemical-rich fruits and vegetables (see Chapters 2 and 8), divide your shopping chores into two parts. Find a farmer's market, food cooperative, or a fruit and vegetable store, and save money while buying the freshest fruits and vegetables possible. Later do the supermarket shopping, looking for the best deals on nonfood items and canned or fresh frozen fruits and vegetables.

Whether you shop at a supermarket or the corner vegetable market, you'll save time and money and make healthier choices if you plan ahead. Decide which meals you will be cooking during the week, check out the menus, and make a grocery list of the items you need.

To speed the shopping process, do it when the vegetable stores or supermarkets are less crowded. The worst time to shop is after 5:00 P.M., right after most people get off work. The markets are crowded with tired, grumpy people. You'll be tired, also. When you are fatigued, it becomes more difficult to avoid the temptation of tasty but unhealthful high-fat or high-sugar foods. Try to shop at a familiar market or store where you know the location of your favorite healthful foods and can skip the long aisles of fat-producing cookies, cakes, and high-sugar cereals (don't forget the oatmeal, though!).

WHAT FOODS TO BUY AND WHY

FRUIT

Fresh fruits of all kinds are good sources of antioxidants, phytochemicals and fiber. Cantaloupes, cranberries, currants, grapefruit, guava, kiwi fruit, oranges, mandarin oranges, mangoes, melons, papaya, pineapples, strawberries, starfruit, and tangerines are good sources of vitamin C. Apricots, cantaloupes, nectarines, persimmons, and papaya are good sources of beta-carotene. Although fresh fruits contain more phytochemical/antioxidant nutrients than processed foods, you may also choose to buy some canned and/or frozen fruit. Avoid canned or frozen fruit with added sugar. Select canned or fresh frozen fruit packed in water or its own juice. Avoid those fruit products that are packed in sugared or "heavy" syrup. Avoid buying packaged fruit. The packaging may disguise rotten spots.

Selecting and Storing Fresh Fruit to Protect
Their Antioxidant Levels

You can make your own fruit-ripening "bowl" by using a toothpick to poke holes in a plastic bag. The holes permit air movement, but the bag contains the fruit gases that hasten ripening.

Remember your mother's old-fashioned thumping test? When trying to determine whether a watermelon or cantaloupe is fresh, put your thumb and index finger together and flick your index finger (as if you were shooting a paper wad when you were in elementary school), thumping the finger against the melon. If you hear a low "plunk," it is fresh. If you hear a higher-toned "plink," it isn't.

Squeeze papayas gently. If they are fresh, they should be soft.

A sure sign that an apple is ripe is a light green color at the bottom of the fruit. Bananas should be slightly green, as they quickly ripen at room temperature. If you want to eat or cook with bananas later that day, buy a small bunch of yellow-skinned ones for immediate use and save the green ones to eat later in the week.

Although relatively high in fat (up to 30 percent of their calories come from fat), avocados are antioxidant-rich and contain certain protective monounsaturated oils. Commonly thought of as a vegetable, avocados are fruits. They should be purchased fresh, but if you're going to cook them later in the week, choose those that still have time to ripen. You can determine whether an avocado is ripe by sticking a toothpick into the stem end. If it slides in and out easily, the avocado is ready to eat.

When shopping for grapes or berries, examine the container bottoms. If they are wet or stained, too much of the fruit is probably mushy or even moldy. Select only those that have dry bottoms.

When selecting oranges, remember that the sweetest have the biggest navel holes. If they feel light in weight, puffy, or spongy, don't buy them. They won't be juicy. Don't be misled by the intensity of their orange color. Most oranges are dyed to make them look tastier. Surprising, those with brown spots, as long as the skins aren't soft or mushy, are the ripest and best to eat. If you want the juiciest grapefruit, look for those with thin skins.

Kiwi fruit is harvested when it is still hard, and most should still feel hard at the time of purchase. They ripen well at room temperature or can be kept in the refrigerator, where they can take weeks to slowly ripen.

VEGETABLES

Fresh vegetables, especially eaten raw, are also excellent sources of antioxidants, phytochemicals, and fiber. Raw vegetables taste good, too, and make great in-between-meal snacks. Good sources of antioxidants and phytochemicals are broccoli, Brussels sprouts, cabbage, carrots, green and red peppers, potatoes, pumpkin, spinach, kale, turnip and other greens, snow peas, sweet potatoes, tomatoes, and winter squash.

Because of their higher phytochemical/antioxidant levels, we highly recommend using fresh vegetables rather than canned or even fresh frozen vegetables whenever possible. Still, we realize that canned or fresh frozen veggies can be stored longer and are convenient for folks who don't like to shop every week. Here's a warning, though: If you buy canned or frozen vegetables, choose those with the lowest sodium and sugar levels. Check food labels. Read the food labels to also check out how much salt (sodium) and sugar has been added. Avoid frozen vegetables packed in high-calorie sugars, creams, or cheese sauces. You can spice up fresh frozen plain vegetables yourself. We will tell you how in the cooking section later in this chapter. It's fun to experiment with various spices.

Selecting and Storing Vegetables

Fresh vegetables should be stored in plastic bags, but unlike those for fruit, the plastic bags don't need to be perforated. The vegetables will retain their moisture and stay fresh longer in unholed plastic bags. It is best to keep most vegetables in the produce crisper section of your refrigerator. The process of overripening and "running" is slowed by refrigeration.

If you are going to cook vegetables right away, a good way to save money is to purchase those that are a day or two old if there are only a few blemishes (oxidation at work again). It's easy to cut away the blemished sections before cooking these vegetables. To freshen blemished or wilted vegetables, after cutting off the brown spots, sprinkle the vegetables with cold water, wrap in paper towels, and put them in the refrigerator for an hour or more.

Remember that fresh vegetables in season are quite a bit cheaper than canned or frozen vegetables.

If you are not going to use them right away, purchase unripened tomatoes. They ripen well at room temperature if kept away from direct sunlight. Ripe tomatoes should be stored in the refrigerator to slow the loss of vitamin C.

Beans and Peas

Beans are low in fat and high in fiber and phytochemicals. Some beans, like green and yellow snap beans, contain the antioxidant vitamin C. Beans and peas, because they are low in fat, high in fiber, and contain phytochemicals, provide protection against cancer and heart disease and are good for our digestive health. Beans also contain more protein per penny than any other food. Many varieties of beans provide B-complex vitamin components, which boost immunity (especially vitamins B_6 and C) and which pregnant women should take to prevent birth defects. Dried beans and peas take a certain amount of preparation. A nutritious alternate is canned beans, which can be rapidly heated or easily added to soups, stews, and casseroles. Try to choose canned beans without large amounts of added meat or fat. Surprising, although "pork and beans" sound high in fat and calories, the amount of added fat in many brands is minimal because such a small amount of pork is added. Bush's Vegetarian Beans, for example, contain 110 calories and fewer than 1 g of fat per serving, while Bush's Deluxe Pork and Beans contain only 13 more calories and 1 g of fat per serving.

Any variety of dried beans or peas can be used to make delicious soups or main entrées. Some of our favorite beans are as follows:

• Baby limas are eaten most often as a side dish, or in soups and casseroles, particularly succotash. Limas are respectable sources of protein, magnesium, and potassium and offer good amounts of thiamine and folate, both components of the B vitamin complex. A lack of folate can cause birth defects. A hearty cup will supply almost two-thirds of a pregnant woman's need for folate; 400 mcg is recommended to prevent birth defects.

• Black beans are often eaten as a main dish with rice because these two foods contain the necessary amino acids that, when combined, form complete protein. They contain good amounts of folate and thiamine. Women who suffer from iron-deficiency-caused anemia should eat black beans with other foods high in vitamin C to maximize iron absorption. Black beans are a great food for people who want to lose weight, since they are heavy with fiber and thus digest slowly, suppressing appetite for hours.

• Chickpeas (also called garbanzo beans), are, because of their nutty taste and firm texture, often used in salads and to make humus, a Middle East seasoned paste. Chickpeas are a good source for folate, contain higher-than-average amounts of vitamin B_6, which also is recommended for women who are pregnant and take oral contraceptives.

• Lentils, which resemble split peas in both looks and use, are eaten most often as a side dish or in soups, stews, and casseroles. They are excellent sources of folate (179 mcg per half cup) and are rich in iron, thiamine, magnesium, and potassium. Like other legumes, they are rich in fiber.

• Pintos are used in Mexican and South American recipes and in soup. They provide good amounts of iron, B vitamins, and, like limas, have two-thirds of a pregnant woman's daily need for folate.

SOUPS

It's best to make your own broth-based soup such as minestrone, chicken and rice, chicken noodle, or vegetable soups, because canned soups can be high in sodium. However, the hectic pace of modern life makes it difficult to create homemade soups. You don't have to go without these appetizing foods. Most stores now also stock low-sodium versions of these soups. Soup before dinner is an excellent idea, especially if you have a weight problem. Studies have shown that people who eat as little as a cup of soup before eating the rest of their lunch or dinner actually ingest fewer overall calories. Naturally we recommend that you stay away from creamy soups or soups made from a gravy base, as these are too high in fat and calories.

BEVERAGES

Green tea, hot or iced, is your best choice.

Soy milk is an excellent drink rich in phytochemicals and low in fat and cholesterol. Other good beverage choices include 1 percent or skim milk, 100 percent fruit juices, vegetable juices, and water. If you like carbonation, unsweetened club soda, mineral water, or seltzers are better for you than diet soda. Coauthor Breecher often mixes and enjoys a half-and-half mixture of cold water and bottled carbonated water.

Use coffee and diet sodas in moderation (no more than two or three servings daily) and stay away from sweetened soda pop. Alcoholic spirits furnish zero nutrients, but studies show that wine in moderation (no more than seven glasses per week for women, 10 to 14 for men) may, perhaps because of the phytochemicals in the grapes, provide some protection against heart disease.

BREADS, CEREALS, AND CRACKERS

Cereals and wheat or oat bran muffins are good sources of fiber and complex carbohydrates, but watch out for the fats or sugar they may contain. Breads, rolls, and muffins or one-half-cup portions of cereal should have 2 g or less of fat and 5 grams or less of sugar per serving. Choose breads of all types including buns, bagels, English muffins, and pita pockets from a 100% whole grain (not just wheat flour) which should be listed as the first ingredient on the package.

EATING OUT

You can make healthy choices for yourself by studying the menu instead of automatically ordering your favorite meal. For instance, at breakfast, skip biscuits, gravy, fried eggs, and bacon or sausage. Instead, order oatmeal or some other high-fiber cereal, whole wheat toast, an English muffin, bagel, or fruit. At any meal, carefully check out the menu and avoid ordering foods high in sugar or fat. Don't be afraid to ask questions about how the food is normally prepared. Avoid fried, battered, creamed, stuffed, scalloped, au gratin, or dishes served with sauce or gravy. Frying doubles the calorie count. Even worse are breaded, fried foods. They are nutritional disasters. The breading soaks up fat like a sponge. Start with a noncream-based soup or salad. Ask the server to bring you a low-calorie dressing on the side. Don't be shy about making special requests, especially at restaurants you regularly patronize. For instance, you can ask for a vegetable plate, or whether other items on the menu, such as fresh fruit or skim milk, are available. You can order fish boiled instead of fried. If you let the management know that you are going to be a regular customer, they will order special foods for you.

After the meal is served, you have choices. You don't have to eat the cuisine just as it is served. You can scrape the skin off the chicken or turkey and trim the fat from a lean steak or prime rib. Go easy on the butter and rolls, and avoid foods heavy with sauces. If you couldn't resist ordering a dish made with a heavy gravy or cream, spoon off most of those high-calorie substances and you can still enjoy the flavor of what remains. Remember, you control how much salad dressing or how many rolls or pieces of bread to eat, and how much butter to use on them. Less is better than more.

WHAT YOU CAN DO NOW

- Before going food shopping, photocopy the sections of this chapter titled "Shopping Made Easy," and "What Foods to Buy and Why." Underline or otherwise highlight the suggestions that will be particularly useful to you on your shopping trip.
- Before eating out, photocopy or at least review the section of this chapter titled "Eating Out." These suggestions can help you refrain from high-calorie choices while enjoying a healthy meal.

TO SUM UP

We have learned that it is possible to eat healthy meals whether you cook at home or eat out. The secret is planning. Plan what you are going to purchase at the supermarket or vegetable store. When you eat out, be mindful of your choices.

Bon appétit!

12

GETTING STARTED AND KEEPING GOING

You can enjoy life while practicing healthy behaviors. Actually, healthy behaviors help you enjoy life. Think about it. It is difficult to enjoy life when you are sick. The fact that you are reading this book shows that you have a deep desire to take the steps necessary to achieve better health. Desire, though, isn't enough. There is a difference between simply desiring better health and being committed to achieve it. One of the most important parts of this program is motivation—getting started and keeping going on this plan.

MOTIVATION IS ESSENTIAL

Your motivation will determine the extent of the personal, active involvement you will invest in this program. Unmotivated readers will fail to heed this advice and may fall victim to premature aging or chronic disease. If you already have health problems or symptoms of premature aging, don't despair. It's never too late to start taking better care of yourself. If you already have a health problem, you have more reason than ever to begin this program. It is a type of motivation known as "instrumental motivation." You have a practical need for heeding the advice in this book. You want to rid yourself of symptoms and feel better.

Those of you who haven't already suffered the adverse effects of poor health may to some degree have a harder time maintaining the effort necessary to make this program work. Knowledge about how to stoke the fires of motivation will be especially useful to you. To become self-motivated, you have to consciously decide and constantly reaffirm that the steps you will be taking to maintain your good health are worthwhile. But watch out: It's easy to become blasé about good health. Don't take it for granted. Premature aging and poor health can sneak up on you.

Psychological research reveals that motivation consists of several elements, desire being only the first of four. Three other components for success include first establishing your goal—in your case realistically deciding on whatever is optimal health for you; developing a positive, "can do" attitude toward the antiaging advice in this book; and last but, as the old cliché states, "certainly not least," effortful behavior on your part to achieve the twin goals of preventing premature aging and achieving better health.

To achieve these twin goals, you need to move and take action. The word *motivation* comes from the Latin term meaning "to move." Another word for movement is action. Action transforms desire into goal achievement. For instance, have you been reading this book with a pencil, pen, or one of those colored markers, taking notes or highlighting points made that directly affect you? Have you started a list of phytochemical- and antioxidant-rich foods to purchase? Have you already purchased those foods, or have you scheduled time to do so? Have you started walking and doing the recommended upper-body exercises? If you haven't taken these steps for your own health, please do so after reading the rest of this chapter.

ADVICE ON HOW TO KEEP GOING

If you have been taking those steps, good for you! You should be experiencing positive benefits. If not, reread this book to determine if you are really putting its recommendations into practice. Remember to reread or to at least skim this book every month or so to check whether you are still doing what you need to do to maintain your personal antiaging program.

Be prepared for setbacks or derailments. Don't give up this program too easily or too quickly. Stay with it long enough to see that it really works. If you have backslid and stopped doing some essential element of this program—exercise, for instance—don't waste time on self-recrimination. Just begin again. For a longer, healthier, more energetic and productive life, the effort is worth it.

Chapter 14 gives you specific steps, such as buying the phytochemical and antioxidant supplements you need to make this program work, but before turning there, let's talk some more about "keeping going" after you have gotten started on this program.

THE IMPORTANCE OF "SELF-TALK"

For long-term motivation, you must become excited about the idea of maintaining good health or achieving what for you is your optimal state of health. Psychology tells us that a powerful way to remain motivated and excited about something is to talk to yourself about it. The way you speak or think about this program will affect your ability to maintain motivation and be successful at it. The belief that the way you speak to yourself and think affects self-motivation has been explored by many behavioral scientists, including Alfred Adler, Albert Ellis, Karen Horney, and Arnold Lazarus. You might enjoy reading their books, which have become classics in the field. (See the notes at the back of this book.)

You talk to yourself during much of your waking day. Your internal monologue is very important in determining how you view yourself and the world around you. It colors your interpretation of all sorts of situations and can determine how you behave in response to many different events. For instance, you now know you should walk about twelve miles per week. But what happens in winter when it rains or snows and becomes frigid for days at end? You could tell yourself that the weather is stopping you from exercising outside. But what about telling yourself that you can go to a fitness center, gym, or even a mall? Many indoor shopping malls let people in several hours before the stores open so that the people can walk inside heated facilities. Of course, you could tell yourself, "It's too much trouble to drive to the fitness center, gym, or mall." That's why it is important to self-monitor what you are telling yourself. When you find that you are giving yourself negative messages, replace them with positive ones.

Proper self-talk can be learned. You can learn to reframe negative situations and look at and speak of them positively. The easiest way to identify a negative message is to ask these three questions:

1. Exactly what am I thinking or saying to myself?
2. Is thinking this way good for my health?
3. Is this thought factual? Is it verifiable or even true?

If you can answer "yes" to questions two and three, it is likely that your self-talk is rational, positive, and health-affirming. If, however, you answer "no" to any of these questions, then you need to eliminate the negative, self-defeating thought. The best way to eliminate a negative thought is to *replace it with a rational, positive thought.* Often the replacement thought will be the direct opposite of the negative, unhealthy one. Let's get back to our exercise example. So what if it is raining or snowing? Instead of saying "I can't," tell yourself "I can" and figure out a way to incorporate exercise into your day. If you can't get out of the house to go to a fitness center, gym, or mall, tell yourself, "I can do my exercises at home." You can walk in place or march from room to room. Also, if you can afford it, our exercise chapter contains suggestions about relatively inexpensive but effective home exercise machines.

VISUALIZATION TO STRENGTHEN MOTIVATION

Another way of maintaining motivation is to practice creating positive pictures in your mind. Building a positive, healthy picture of self in your mind is an important motivational tool. If you can see yourself as aging gracefully while in good health, it will help you begin and maintain the process of accomplishing that goal.

Here's some background. Some of us think in words, others think in terms of images. Most of us combine the two modes, depending on the situation. In fact, as young children most of us probably learned to think in terms of images first, before we learned to talk. Now that we are blessed with language, we often forget our innate ability to process thoughts in the form of images. Yet scientists tell us that visual thought is an extremely powerful method of learning and can be a very effective tool for positive motivational self-programming. Champions of all types already know this. For example, in his book *Golf My Way,* Jack Nicklaus wrote: "I never hit a shot, not even in practice, without having a sharp, in-focus picture in my head. First, I'd 'see' the ball where I wanted it to finish. . . . Then, I 'see' the ball going there . . . the next scene shows me making the kind of swing that will turn the previous images into reality."

You, too, can learn to create vivid, self-motivating images. Follow these directions. Sit on a cozy couch or chair wearing loose, comfortable clothing. Close your eyes and take several deep, calming breaths. Recall a pleasant memory. Take your time. Enjoy the scene.

Welcome back. Now ask yourself:

1. Did I visualize vivid, clear images?
2. Were the images in color?
3. Did the images move? Did the action in my imaged scene unwind like a movie with continuous action, or were the images more like a series of snapshots?
4. Was I an observer? Did I watch myself perform as I would watch an actor or actress in a movie? Or, during the visualization, did I experience myself as a participant in the action?
5. How intense was my participation? Did I feel like I was reliving the scene?

By answering these questions and practicing the technique you can learn to manipulate your self-created images as positive health reinforcers. You are the director of this "movie" in your mind. Your "camera" is your "mind's eye." You are the one who decides to use color or black-and-white film, or whether to use slides or videotape. For instance, did you see the scene in black-and-white? Next time, try adding color. Was your pleasant image a snapshot or a movie? If it was a snapshot, next time try to add movement. Change the image in your mind from a photo or series of photos to a motion picture. You control the depth of field, the focus, the duration of the "camera" shot, and scores of other variables.

Always practice this exercise using pleasant memories. After you have practiced and become skillful at using the technique, try your newfound visualization skills to picture yourself as aging gracefully, in good physical and mental health. Some researchers actually teach this technique to cancer patients to use to combat their malignancies. Their research is intriguing but far from conclusive. However, as a motivational tool, self-visualization cannot be beat.

THE RESPONSIBILITY INSIGHT

Adding healthy years to your life is a worthwhile goal, but you are the only one who can take the steps to accomplish it. Life becomes easier when you accept the responsibility to take disciplined actions to enhance your own health. Acknowledge that whatever health level you are at today is a result of decisions (eating high-fat foods, for example) and actions (smoking, for instance) or inactions (for example, failure to exercise) that you took in the past. If you want your future years to be long and healthy, it is up to you to change any self-defeating "self-talk" and resulting inappropriate behaviors to positive affirmations and responsible action.

WHAT YOU CAN DO NOW

- Establish your goal. Write it down.
- Cultivate a positive "can do" attitude by writing a set of positive self-talk affirmations such as "I make time in my day for exercise," "I enjoy healthy foods," and "I make time for healthful behaviors during the day."

- Take action. Don't just read the above statements; move on them.
- Monitor your "self-talk." Use the three questions in the section "The Importance of 'Self-Talk'" in this chapter to identify any negative messages you may be sending to yourself. Replace them with positive, rational ones.

TO SUM UP

- We have learned that the desire to enjoy good health isn't enough. You have to be committed to achieve it.
- You can light the fires of motivation—and get started and keep going on this program—by using the self-talk and visualization techniques explained in this chapter.
- The program does take a small commitment of time. For a longer, healthier, and more productive life, the effort is worth it.
- No one can do it for you. You have the tools and knowledge needed to live longer and healthier. It is your responsibility to make the correct decisions and take the proper actions to ensure your good health.

13

MELATONIN UPDATE

MELATONIN: MIRACLE HORMONE, NATURAL WONDER DRUG, PROMISING ANTIOXIDANT—OR JUST A FAD?

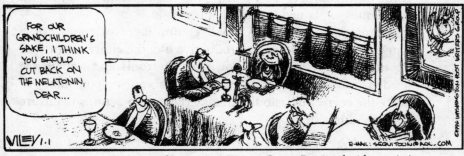

Non Sequitor cartoon © 1996 Washington Post Writers Group. Reprinted with permission.

Newsweek hailed melatonin as one of the "hottest pills of the decade."[1] Hundreds of thousands of individuals are taking it. Pharmacies and health food stores at first couldn't keep up with the demand. Source Naturals, one of the largest wholesalers of the hormone, sold 1 million bottles in 1994 and claims sales of approximately 7 million bottles in 1995.

People are excited about melatonin because of the many and various health claims made on its behalf. Until the 1990s, many of melatonin's benefits to humans—let alone its mechanisms of action—remained shrouded in mystery. Today, to use the words of a 1995

Science News article, "scientists have variously described its primary role as the regulator of the body's internal clock, a defense against biologically damaging free radicals, an age-retarding chemical, a trigger for sleep, and a coordinator of the hormones involved in fertility."[2] No wonder so many people are buying and using it as a supplement.

Many of the claims made on melatonin's behalf are controversial, but many others have been supported. For instance, its effectiveness as a sleep inducer is well documented. While its uses as an antiaging drug and as a biorhythm regulator remain controversial, it may indeed be a life extender. Evidence is mounting about its protective effects as an antioxidant against heart disease and cancer. Claims that melatonin can prevent the onset of Alzheimer's disease, relieve asthma, and prevent diabetes and Down's syndrome while also helping victims of migraines, epilepsy, autism, balding, schizophrenia, Parkinson's disease, and Sudden Infant Death syndrome are premature, but research in these areas appears promising. "Melatonin could play a significant protective role in both the initial as well as the progressive stages of many diseases," says Dr. Russel J. Reiter, a cellular biologist and author of the December 1995 Bantam hardcover book *Melatonin: Your Body's Natural Wonder Drug,* coauthored with Jo Robinson.[3]

Let's look at some of the evidence, medical research that relates to these claims:

- There's good evidence for melatonin's effectiveness as a sleep inducer and some evidence that it can soften the effects of jet lag.
- Whether melatonin can delay or reverse the ravages of aging is more controversial, but it can extend some people's lives, especially those with family histories or other risk factors for heart disease or cancer.
- Even the claims that melatonin may delay or prevent the onset of Alzheimer's disease and other diseases have promise.

EVIDENCE OF MELATONIN'S ROLE AS A SLEEPING AID

Melatonin is a hormone produced by the pineal gland. That organ was so named because of its pine conelike shape. The pineal gland is a reddish-gray organ the size of a pea in the middle of the back portion of the human brain. For many years physiologists thought that the pineal gland was as irrelevant to modern humans as the appendix. We now know that this gland secretes melatonin in a rhythmic fashion throughout the day. Melatonin production is stimulated by darkness and thus is elevated at night. When melatonin levels are high, people feel sleepy. However, as we age, melatonin production dramatically decreases. Thus older people tend to experience insomnia more than younger people.

There's good news for both the older and the younger insomniacs.

THE GOOD NEWS FOR OLDER INSOMNIACS

According to the September 1995 issue of the medical journal *Sleep,* in what was described as the "first published report of the therapeutic effect of melatonin in older people,"[4] Israeli researchers found that supplements of that hormone can help elderly insomniacs fall asleep faster and stay asleep longer. The study consisted of three one-week treatment periods with two-week breaks in between. The insomniacs took capsules containing either 2 mg of fast- or slow-release melatonin or an identical-looking but inactive placebo two hours before their desired bedtime. It was a double-blind study—until the study was complete, neither the participants nor the researchers knew which insomniacs were getting the various types of melatonin or placebo during each of the three one-week study periods. During the entire study, the participants wore miniaturized sleep-recording devices. The recordings later told researchers how long the participants took to fall asleep and how long and how rest-fully they slept. When the initial study was complete, it was found that while the fast-release melatonin influenced the speed of falling asleep, the slow- or sustained-release melatonin made sleep more restful. A follow-up study in which seventeen of the twenty-six vol-unteers took 1 mg of slow-release melatonin for two months showed that even at the reduced dosage, over time, the insomniacs fell asleep faster and slept better.

The Israeli researchers weren't the first to publish results about the benefits of melatonin in aiding the sleep of elderly people. That honor may belong to three English authors. Writing in an August 1995 article in the prestigious British medical journal *Lancet,* a team of researchers led by Dr. D. Garfinkel described a similar random-ized, double-blind, crossover study in which twelve elderly men aged sixty-eight to eighty-four, took either 2 mg per night of time-release melatonin or a placebo for three weeks. The way the study was designed, all the subjects took both melatonin and a placebo in different three-week periods, not knowing which time period they were on the pineal hormone. The results, according to *Lancet:* "Sleep efficiency was significantly greater after melatonin than after placebo. . . . Melatonin deficiency may have an important role in the high frequency of insomnia among elderly people. Controlled-re-lease melatonin replacement therapy effectively improves sleep quality in this population." These findings add to the growing body of evidence showing that melatonin plays an important role in reg-ulating sleep.[5]

THE GOOD NEWS FOR YOUNGER INSOMNIACS

An earlier study of melatonin's sleep-enhancing effects on younger men, published in a 1994 issue of the journal *Proceedings of the Na-tional Academy of Sciences,* revealed that those who took a small dose of melatonin fell asleep within about six minutes and slept longer than after they were given a placebo. This study was duplicated by Dr. Richard J. Wurtman, professor of neuroscience at the Massachu-setts Institute of Technology (MIT). Dr. Wurtman and his colleagues reported in the May 1995 issue of *Clinical Pharmacology and Therapeutics* that a dose one-eight-hundredth of that given in earlier studies "induces sleep without side effects." Unlike hypnotic sleeping pills, melatonin does not alter the "normal architecture" of sleep, including the timing and duration of dream phases characterized by rapid eye movement. "This compound produces natural sleep," concludes Dr. Wurtman. "The data suggest that very tiny doses" (as little as 0.1 mg) can combat insomnia. Dr. Ray Sahelian of Los Angeles, author of the book *Melatonin: Nature's Sleeping Pill,* says, "I think eventually melatonin will make prescription sleeping pills all but obsolete."[6]

JET LAG

The pineal gland was considered the "seat of the soul" by early Greek philosophers, but modern researchers believe that the gland works as a "pacemaker" or "biological clock," regulating our bodies' metabolic processes from sunrise to sunset. Thus, as medical writer Joseph Anthony pointed out in a November 1995 article in *American Health,* it was "a short jump from melatonin as a natural sleeping pill" to studies on its effectiveness as a treatment for jet lag. The reasoning was that since melatonin taken in the daytime induces sleepiness in most people, it can help reset the body's internal clock after a long jet flight when the traveler arrives in the morning and finds himself or herself groggy but unable to sleep. Bright light during the day suppresses the natural production of melatonin by the pineal gland, but supplemental melatonin may make up for the lack of natural melatonin in jet-lagged travelers. Researchers have shown that a "brief nightly regimen of 5 mg can help airline workers adjust to new time zones," according to an August 1995 *Newsweek* article.

BENEFITS TO SHIFT WORKERS

Employees whose jobs require them to switch shifts periodically often complain of fatigue and insomnia. Periodic shift changes often disrupt the circadian rhythm, also known as the sleep/wake cycle, of workers. If you are a shift worker starting a new shift that you will be on for four weeks or more, consider using melatonin to help you adjust to your sleep pattern. Take 1.5 to 3 mg at least one-half hour before the new time when you want to fall asleep. After several days you may be able to "trick" your body into thinking it is time to sleep during a time period in which it was used to being awake.

PERSONAL EXPERIENCES OF THE AUTHORS ON MELATONIN

JIM'S DIARY

I have been taking one-half of a 3 mg tablet of melatonin nightly since September of 1995. I don't normally have trouble falling asleep, but felt that with all the publicity that melatonin was getting and because of its antioxidant effects, I should try it. At first I took a full 3 mg tablet each night. As usual I slept soundly, but upon awakening I felt groggy. It was the same feeling I had experienced after the rare occasions in the past when I felt unusually stressed and to ensure a good night's sleep had taken either 25 mg of Benadryl (the antihistamine diphenylhydramine that in some people but not others causes drowsiness) or 2.5 mg of diazepam, the generic name for the prescription drug Valium. I remembered the "morning-after groggy feeling" of those drugs. I felt the same way on the morning after the 3 mg dose of melatonin. So I decreased my melatonin dose to one-half tablet (1.5 mg in my case) every evening. Since then I have slept well, and the feeling of grogginess went away.

To test the effects of jet lag, I took melatonin nightly during my two-week trip to China in October 1995. I didn't take it on the jet plane because I was traveling alone and did not want to experiment with a substance as powerful as melatonin, even though there have been popular and scientific reports that melatonin is *not* toxic in large doses over short spans of time. Upon arriving in China I started taking either 1.5 mg or 3 mg tablets every night, depending on how stimulated I felt by the day's activities. Regardless of the dose, I slept wonderfully and felt well rested. I had the energy to climb the famous Great Wall of China while younger friends waited at the bottom. I raced a forty-five-year-old Japanese lady professor to the top of a nine-story shrine and a thirty-eight-year-old California student to the top of the mountain and won both times.

Still, I am not sure that melatonin is actually a wonder drug. I have taken it for four months and have seen some favorable effects but no adverse ones. It is a better sleep aid than diphenylhydramine or diazepam. However, I may be a little more assertive or pushy than usual, so perhaps after four months melatonin is exerting a subtle effect on my behavior. I'll give you a personal update when I autograph your book.

MAURY'S DIARY

I have a medical condition known as sleep apnea and have suffered from related insomnia for years. My sleeping patterns have been erratic and unrestful. I started taking melatonin a couple of months before Dr. Anderson. At first I took a 2.5 mg tablet sublingually (under the tongue). Five to ten minutes after it melted, my eyelids became heavy and I was able to sleep and dream comfortably throughout the night. However, at this dose, like Jim I had a hard time getting going in the mornings. So I dropped the dose drastically. I now take a small bite out of the tablet, probably no more than 0.5 mg. Naturally, after several nights of such bites the remaining tablet crumbles. Still, I usually get three restful nights of sleep from one tablet. What a deal! Based on my experience and the medical studies I have examined, I think melatonin is a superb sleep aid.

I haven't been flying to China and climbing mountains, but possibly because my sleep patterns have changed, I do feel more energetic. Indeed, friends and relatives have noticed and remarked about my increased energy levels. I can't ascribe this beneficial change just to melatonin. Since I am an insulin-dependent diabetic, I have been taking Dr. Anderson's antioxidant, antiaging health program advice at the disease-reversal level. So naturally I feel more energetic.

MELATONIN'S POTENTIAL TO EXTEND LIVES AND FIGHT DISEASE

The most important cells of the pineal gland are called pinealocytes. It is these cells that produce and secrete melatonin. However, the secretion of melatonin by the pineal gland has been shown to decline progressively as we age. The progressive decrease in the number of pinealocytes as we age may be the cause of the age-related reduction in melatonin production. People over age sixty secrete 80% less melatonin than twenty-year-olds. A two-year-old normally has a high blood serum level of 350 units of melatonin per 100 ml, while a ninety-year-old has levels below 30 units per 100 ml. This dramatic drop has important ramifications. Deficiencies of melatonin are thought to be involved in the aging process. For one thing, if the body secretes less melatonin, there are fewer antioxidant defenders to protect our systems from the ravages of free radicals.

Some scientists have theorized that a deficiency of melatonin may be a critical starting point for a wide range of degenerative diseases. For instance, Alzheimer's disease patients have been found to have abnormally low melatonin levels. The dementia associated with Alzheimer's disease is probably, at least in part, caused by free radical destruction of brain cells. This leads to the hope that the intake of supplemental melatonin can protect against such degenerative changes. There is reason to believe that melatonin can achieve this. Research suggests that supplemental melatonin may protect against effects of free-radical-induced brain cell damage. Prestigious researchers call melatonin "the most potent and effective [free radical] . . . scavenger yet discovered."[7]

Melatonin also has natural anticancer properties, including the ability to enhance the immune system's killer cells. It has been observed that when melatonin levels are low, the body becomes more prone to cancer. Decreased melatonin levels have been associated with breast and prostate cancer, melanoma, and malignancies of the ovaries. Laboratory studies have shown positive results against breast cancer by reducing the number of tumor-producing estrogen receptor sites and the sizes of tumors. In a few human clinical trials, melatonin has been combined experimentally with Tamoxifen, an estrogen inhibitor. While these preliminary studies are encouraging, researchers have a long way to go to prove that melatonin alone inhibits the initiation, progression, and transformation of cancer cells. (Please review Chapter 4 for our explanation of the cancer process.) There also are few or no studies at this time that show melatonin reduces risks for heart disease. Based on our understanding of the medical literature, we believe that there is much less persuasive literature and support for melatonin's beneficial effects on cancer and heart disease than there is, for instance, on the beneficial effects of soy isoflavones for those conditions (see Chapter 7, "The Joys of Soy").

SOME CAVEATS ABOUT MELATONIN

The highly respected and reliable *Medical Letter* reviewed melatonin research and in its November 24, 1995 issue concluded that "Melatonin might turn out to be an effective hypnotic and could have some beneficial effect on jet lag, but large, controlled trials in jet travelers and patients with insomnia have not been done . . . the adverse effects of taking the hormone are unknown."[8]

The *Medical Letter* also raises the question of the purity of the melatonin being sold. As *Newsweek* explained in its November 6, 1995, issue, "The FDA monitors drugmakers' raw materials and production methods, but because melatonin is sold as a 'dietary supplement,' it isn't subject to such scrutiny."[9] Of course, the same can be said about countless products sold "over-the-counter" and in nutrition stores.

Still, I, Dr. Anderson, do not recommend the long-term use of melatonin because studies on that substance's long-term effects have not been done. According those that have, it appears *not to be toxic even at large amounts for short periods of time.* In my personal experience, it certainly produced fewer side effects than the antihistamine diphenylhydramine. However, unlike that cold-symptom reliever, melatonin hasn't had the benefit of years and years of scientific research on humans. No one knows whether high doses of melatonin, even though they cause no immediate harm, might have long-term effects or whether those effects will be beneficial or harmful.

As a physician, that makes me uncomfortable. Melatonin is widely available at health food stores and pharmacies and can be purchased and taken as easily as Life Savers. While it is true that many drugs prescribed by doctors have more side effects than melatonin on a short-term basis, at least the patients are monitored by their physicians.

I agree with Dr. Reiter, who identified categories of persons who should *not* take melatonin, in his book *Melatonin: Your Body's Natural Wonder Drug.* They include children, people taking steroid drugs such as cortisone, prednisone, and dexamethasone; pregnant women or women wanting to conceive; nursing mothers; people with severe mental illness or severe allergies; people with autoimmune diseases such as rheumatoid arthritis or lupus; and people with immune-system cancers such as lymphoma or leukemia.

Melatonin proponents believe that its long-term effects will be beneficial and life-extending. Skeptics focus on possible unknown dangers. Where do I stand? If you are a risk taker who is very concerned about aging or degenerative diseases such as Alzheimer's and you don't fall into one of the above groups, you might want to take melatonin on the chance that it will slow down the aging process and delay the occurrence of degenerative brain diseases. The potential benefits are good—I wouldn't say "excellent" at this point—and the potential risks are small—not minuscule, but small.

TO SUM UP

- Melatonin is an effective sedative and aid to sleep. With the proper dose, it will help many people get a good night's sleep.
- Melatonin may reduce problems with jet lag. It has minimal short-term side effects and is certainly worth trying.
- In animal studies, under certain unusual conditions, melatonin dramatically slows down the aging process. The effects of melatonin on aging in humans have not been carefully tested and are unknown.
- Melatonin may slow down conditions such as Alzheimer's disease leading to premature deterioration of the brain. Melatonin's antioxidant properties may protect brain cells from damage.
- The long-term safety of melatonin in humans is unknown. Currently the purity of this hormone is not standardized as for hormones such as thyroid hormone and insulin, so the dose taken from time to time may vary.

WHAT YOU CAN DO NOW

- If you have difficulty sleeping, take 1 mg or 1.5 mg (one-third or one-half of a 3-mg tablet) about an hour before bedtime. Follow the specific guidelines provided by Drs. Pierpaoli and Regelson[10] and Dr. Reiter.[11]
- If you experience major jet lag problems when traveling, take one 3 mg tablet on the evening of your arrival. Take either 1.5 mg or 3 mg nightly for the next week.
- Slow-release forms of melatonin are being developed by reputable drug companies. Watch for these better, standardized, more effective forms of melatonin.

To conclude, melatonin is probably not a fad, but it's not a panacea either. Melatonin is a potent antioxidant, but it is not the only antioxidant. Your best bet for overall good health and an extended life span is to review Table 8.1 in this book and practice the behaviors and get the optimal amounts of antioxidants and phytochemicals through diet and the antioxidant supplements shown there.

14

PUTTING YOUR ANTIOXIDANT, ANTIAGING PLAN TOGETHER

Know that your antioxidant program can do these things:

- help you live longer and healthier;
- reduce your risk for heart attack, stroke, and other circulation problems;
- protect you from a variety of cancers;
- lessen your chances of getting Alzheimer's disease or other deterioration of brain function;
- decrease chances of developing diabetes, skin disease, and certain eye problems.

You are anxious to get started.

Remember you were promised that this required only thirty minutes per day and $10 per week?

Now we come to the nitty-gritty time. Having read Chapter 12, you're motivated and raring to go. You are probably asking yourself, "What is my first step? What do I need to do, and how do I do it?"

Making lifestyle changes are difficult for some people (about 99 percent of us). Consequently we have broken these changes down into baby steps. There is stage 1 (crawling), stage 2 (walking), and stage 3 (running). Move slowly through the stages and learn the skills well before moving on. Remember, toddlers get injured when they try to run before they have mastered walking.

STAGE 1

First: Identify and purchase the right supplements. You can shop for these today and start taking all of them tomorrow, jump-starting your antioxidant program in fewer than twenty-four hours. You will need these:

- *multivitamin and mineral supplement.* Get one—either a capsule or a tablet—that has the RDA (recommend dietary allowance) for most of the vitamins, minerals, and trace elements. Do not include iron unless your doctor has specifically told you that you need iron.
- *antioxidant supplement.* Obtain a combination tablet or capsule (e.g. Protegra, Vitegra, or Procea) that contains beta-carotene, 5000 IU or 3 mg; vitamin C, 250 mg; vitamin E, 200 IU or 200 mg; and selenium, 15 mcg. Take one or two twice daily as recommended in Table 8.1.
- *enteric-coated aspirin.* Take one 325-mg.-tablet daily; buy a bottle of three hundred to last for ten months.
- *fish oil capsules.* If recommended in Table 8.1, take two daily; buy fish oil capsules (such as Max-EPA) that contain 300 mg EPA and 200 mg DHA per 1 g.
- *melatonin.* Optional (see Chapter 13); buy a 3-mg tablet and try half a tablet thirty to sixty minutes before bedtime for sleep or one tablet in the evening to reduce problems with jet lag.
- *Pycnogenol.* Optional (see Table 8.1); try the pycnogenol capsules initially. Take 50 mg every morning. If you tolerate these and feel they are worth the expense, shop around to find a less expensive form.
- *FABB.* Optional (see Table 8.1.); take tablets or combinations to

provide folic acid 1 to 2 mg per day; vitamin B_6 25 to 50 mg per day; vitamin B_{12}, 10 to 25 mcg per day.

Second: Start your walking program.

- Estimate how much you currently are walking; calculate it in minutes or miles.
- Increase your walking by 50 percent. If you currently walk ten minutes, five days per week (fifty minutes per week), increase to fifteen minutes, five or six days per week. If you are walking one mile per day, four days per week (four miles per week), increase to six miles per week.
- Increase your walking by 50 percent every one to two weeks until you are at your goal.
- Remember, the minimum goal (a good level) is six miles of walking per week; a better level is twelve miles per week; and the best level is twenty miles per week. Diligent readers recognize that these levels are lower than in my last book.[1] This new recommendation includes upper-body exercises as summarized in Table 8.1. The total amount of aerobic exercise being recommended is the same as previously.

Third: Begin your food plan.

- Look at Table 8.3. Make one healthy choice at each meal. For breakfast, for example, start drinking tea *or* add fruit juice. For lunch, for example, have vegetable juice or high-antioxidant vegetables (see the honor roll of vegetables in Table 8.2), *or* have an orange or grapes. For the evening meal, for example, have iced tea or vegetable juice (red wine also will give you benefits here), *or* have a vegetable from the honor roll.
- Include at least one high-antioxidant fruit *and* one high-antioxidant vegetable (from the honor roll, Table 8.2) in your diet daily. You can do that.
- Make one other positive nutrition change from Table 8.1. For example, choose one of the following: eat fish twice weekly (broiled, of course); start including soy products in your diet

several times weekly (a nutrition bar is the easiest way to go—I have one daily); use garlic several times weekly; drink two cups of tea daily; eat tree nuts (pecans or walnuts, not peanuts) several times weekly; start purchasing seedless purple grapes and nibbling on them daily; or purchase one can of vegetable juice for use daily.

Fourth: Review the suggestions in the column labeled "Other" in Table 8.1.

- Congratulate yourself on not smoking. For the 10 percent of readers who still smoke, see if you can decrease your number of cigarettes daily, or stop.
- Buckle your seat belts to reduce your risk of serious injury or death by 50 percent (think about your children, grandchildren, and friends who will miss you, or, worse yet, have to take care of you with a severe handicap).
- R&R keep a military force fit, alert, and ready. Getting adequate sleep, quality time with family and friends, getaway weekends, and at least one week of genuine, relaxing vacation yearly are essential to longevity and high quality of life.
- Moderation in alcohol use (one glass of red wine for women and two for men daily) or, preferably from a health standpoint, abstinence; avoiding smoking and drug use; and not being a workaholic are important for health and longevity.

STAGE 2

First: Continue your supplements. Shop around for less expensive brands. Remember, you can do this for fewer than $10 per week.

Second: Start your upper-body exercises. Decide how you best can do this, and sample various types of exercise equipment at exercise shops, discount stores, or fitness centers. Consider purchasing a Cardioglide or E-Force apparatus. Start with five minutes of exercise several days per week, and work up to the level suggested in Table 8.1.

Third: Move to the next level in your food plan. At this level you should be doing two-thirds of the things outlined in Table 8.1.

- *Make two healthy choices at every meal.* For breakfast have tea, choosing either a fruit or a fruit juice that makes the honor roll. For lunch choose a salad or a sandwich bag of vegetables from the honor roll, and have grapes or another antioxidant-rich fruit. For dinner enjoy honor roll vegetables and fruits.
- *Increase the use of soy protein products.* According to the guidelines in Table 8.1. include one to three servings of soy protein daily. You can get your soy in with soy beverage (up to 20 g of soy protein daily from special homemade beverages or commercial beverages containing soy protein isolate from Protein Technology International, St. Louis), soy muffins (3 g of soy protein per muffin), or nutrition bars (mine has 9 g of soy protein). Enjoy tofu stir-fry, tofu spaghetti sauce (see recipe section, Chapter 9), and other tofu dishes.
- *Make one other healthy food choice daily:* Choose one of the following: Eat fish twice weekly; use garlic several times weekly; drink two cups of tea daily; eat tree nuts several times weekly; purchase seedless purple grapes and nibble on them daily; or drink one canful of vegetable juice daily.

Fourth: Maintain the health-promoting habits in Table 8.1. ("Other") and see if you have room for improvement.

STAGE 3

Now you are ready to run with your antioxidant program. Review the goals for your protection level in Table 8.1. At stage 3 you should be meeting or exceeding all the goals outlined in the table.

First: Continue your supplements. Already they are keeping the free radicals from damaging your DNA (see Chapter 2) and protecting you from aging, cancer, and heart attack.

Second: Continue to increase your level of exercise until you meet the goal. While some of you may feel that you cannot achieve a preventive level of walking or physical activity, my experience with thousands of obese patients suggests that you may be able to. See the case of Martha given below.

Third: Increase your selection of antioxidant-rich foods as summarized in Table 8.1, ensuring that you are getting at least five servings of honor roll vegetables and fruits daily. Enjoy soy protein in a wide variety of ways and start taking your family and friends to the Chinese restaurants where you can have braised tofu (in a dry wok without oil). Try tempeh and other forms of soy protein. Become a connoisseur of green tea, and share this information with your friends. Cook with fresh garlic to spice up your foods (to be honest, I usually use minced garlic that comes in a 4-oz jar). Locate the produce market where you can get ripe kiwi, purple grapes, and other fruits all year 'round. Finally, maintain a high fiber intake and a low fat intake to keep your weight at a desirable level.

Fourth: Maintain the "other" health-promoting habits to complement your food program, exercise plan, and antioxidant supplement regimen.

Congratulations. You have graduated from our program and are now authorized to teach others these health-promoting activities.

MARTHA INCREASES HER PHYSICAL ACTIVITY BY 2,500 PERCENT

Recently an obese woman with severe arthritis limiting her to a wheelchair or very slow locomotion with a walker came to our weight-loss program. She had essentially no capacity to exercise. After four months of treatment and a weight loss of fifty pounds she is a very different woman. She went shopping in a mall for the first time in ten years. She went to Branson, Missouri, to see Glen Campbell, her first out-of-town trip in six years. She couldn't exercise when she started, but now she gets the equivalent of twenty miles per week in walking. She, like dozens of my patients with commitment and slow increases in activity, achieved levels of activity that are twenty to fifty times more than previously. Weight loss helps, but slow and steady practice allows virtually all of my patients, up to age ninety years, to achieve preventive levels of physical activity (six miles of walking per week).

APPENDIX A: ANTIOXIDANT AND PHYTOCHEMICAL ADVISORY

My most important recommendations have to do with beta-carotene and vitamins C and E. The most controversial recommendation may be that regarding beta-carotene. While a number of prestigious organizations have recommended 15 to 30 mg daily (in other words, 25,000 to 50,000 IU), many experts are concerned about these levels and are using lower doses in clinical trials. One concern is the yellowing of the skin seen in some women on doses of more than 15 to 18 mg daily. Beta-carotene is the only antioxidant that gives you a protective amount (6 mg) in single servings of antioxidant-rich fruits and vegetables such as apricots and cantaloupe and carrots and sweet potatoes. To get protective amounts of vitamin C you have to eat four to six servings of vitamin C-rich fruit and vegetables. For vitamin E you need forty to one hundred servings to achieve a protection level. That is why I strongly recommend supplements of vitamins C and E. Including 6 to 12 mg of beta-carotene with your supplement is recommended, but optional.

Allium vegetables: See Appendix B.

Alpha-tocopherol: See the vitamin E entry in this appendix.

Antioxidants: A group of elements including enzymes, vitamins, minerals, and other substances that oppose the process of oxidation. (See the oxidation entry in Appendix B.)

Beta-carotene: This vitamin precursor joins vitamins C and E to make the "Big Three" major antioxidant vitamins. Beta-carotene is found in orange vegetables such as sweet potatoes and carrots; green vegetables; and fruits such as cantaloupe, mangoes, peaches, pink grapefruit, and tangerines. It is a precursor of vitamin A, meaning that beta-carotene is converted into vitamin A as the body needs it. Don't confuse beta-carotene with vitamin A, since large doses of vitamin A are toxic, while large doses of beta-carotene are not, because the body converts only the amounts it needs to form vitamin A.

Recommendation: 10,000 IU (6 mg) daily from antioxidant-rich fruits or vegetables or a supplement.

Special needs: Colon cancer is second only to lung cancer as a major cause of death among American males. Some 50,000 females were also diagnosed with colon cancer in a recent year (1994). People with any type of cancer and people with family histories of colon cancer should ingest at least 30,000 IU (18 mg) per day. As outlined in Table 8.1, I recommend a supplement providing 12 mg per day for persons in the tailored protection or disease reversal groups.

Capsicum and capsaicin: See Appendix B.

Carnitine: See L-Carnitine later in this appendix.

Catechins: See Appendix B.

Chromium: The average American diet may be deficient in this essential trace mineral, according to several studies. Chromium is believed to help stabilize blood sugar levels, but claims that it melts off fat have not been supported by adequate research. Chromium is readily available in the North American diet. It is found in beer, brewer's yeast, brown rice, cheese, corn and corn oil, dried beans, whole grains, mushrooms, potatoes, calves' liver, and, in lesser amounts, other meats. Still, studies indicate that 50 percent to 90 percent of the population aren't getting enough chromium, says biochemist Richard Anderson (no relation to Dr. Jim Anderson) at the USDA's Human Nutrition Research Center. That's because chromium is not easily absorbed by the human body. All but 2 percent of the chromium ingested from food is excreted by the body. In a Danish study, people with low blood sugar who exhibited symptoms of chilliness, trembling, and emotional instability reduced those symptoms after taking two tablespoons of brewer's yeast (a rich source of chromium) every day for three months. In another study, this one at the State University of New York at Syracuse, subjects who also took two tablespoonsful of brewer's yeast each day for only two months had significant drops in their blood cholesterol levels.

Recommendation: 150 mcg daily. Chromium picolinate supplements are readily available at pharmacies and health food stores. This form of chromium is "user-friendly"—that is, it is more easily absorbed and used by the body.

Special needs: Persons with adult-onset (Type II) diabetes should ingest at least 200 mcg daily.

Coenzyme Q: This important antioxidant is essential to all human life because it regulates the intake of oxygen to cells, thus supplying the "spark" essential for the cell to produce energy. Coenzyme Q is carried by LDL cholesterol particles. Low levels of this substance allow the LDL to be oxidized by free radicals, leading to hardening to the arteries (see Chapter 3). High levels of this antioxidant protect against free radicals.

Recommendation: No recommendation for general protection. Some authorities recommend preventive doses of 30 mg daily for persons over age fifty.

Special needs: Anyone taking the "statin" family of cholesterol-lowering drugs (fluvastatin or Lescol, lovastatin or Mevacor, pravastatin or Pravacol, or simvastatin or Zocor) should take 30 to 60 mg daily, since these drugs reduce Q-10 levels in LDL particles. Persons with congestive heart failure may benefit from Q-10 intake; the recommended dosage for these people is 120 mg twice daily.

Daidzein: An isoflavone, another important nutrient from soy. See the genistein entry in this appendix.

Garlic: This herb, a member of the allium group of vegetables (see Table 4.1 and Table 8.2), has antioxidant properties and contains important phytochemicals that act to lower blood cholesterol and decrease blood clotting, thus providing protection against heart disease and stroke. Research also indicates that garlic decreases cancer risk.

Recommendation: Eat garlic-containing foods as often as possible.

Special needs: People at risk for heart disease. Persons who wish special protection against heart disease should have at least one clove of garlic, or ¼ teaspoonful of minced garlic, or one garlic tablet (600 mg) four times weekly. People who already have heart disease should eat garlic daily.

Genistein: A soy protein that *may* provide protection against coronary heart disease as well as breast and prostate cancer. The absorption rate and effects of both genistein and daidzein are still unclear; research is continuing. Scientists at the University of Alabama at Birmingham and elsewhere are working on developing a genistein milkshake for men at risk of developing prostate disease. (Men at risk for prostate cancer can be identified if they take a lab test called the prostate-specific antigen.) A similar soy-based product is being developed for women who have had, or are at risk of developing, breast cancer, or who want to use this milder phytoestrogen as estrogen replacement therapy.[1] Soy protein sources rich in genistein—and its sister isoflavone, daidzein—available now include lactose-free soy milk; soy flour; textured soy protein; isolated soy protein; tofu; and tempeh, a chewy soy cake.

Recommendation: One-half to one ounce of soy protein daily should provide adequate amounts of both genistein and daidzein. (See Chapter 7 and Table 8.1.) A goal for preventative protection is to eat seven servings (7 to 10 g per serving) per week.

Special needs: Postmenopausal women who do not take estrogens and those with strong family histories of breast cancer should have at least two 15- to 20-g servings of soy protein per day. People with a diagnosis of breast cancer or heart disease should have three 25- to 30-g servings daily.

Ginkgo biloba: An extract made from the leaves of the oldest tree on earth, ginkgo is touted and used by millions as a brainpower and memory booster. Studies indicate that it is a powerful antioxidant providing beneficial effects in cases of Alzheimer's disease; asthma; circulatory disorders, including impotence, eye problems, headaches, and hemorrhoids; and hearing difficulties, including tinnitus (ringing of the ears).

Recommendation: No recommendation. Some authorities recommend 20 to 40 mg two or three times daily.

Special needs: Because of its potential to preserve brain function, individuals with family histories of Alzheimer's disease or people over age fifty who exhibit a decrease in their short-term memory are advised to take 40 mg two or three times daily. Doses should *not* exceed 160 mg daily.

Ginseng: The ginseng root has been used by Chinese medicine for more than four thousand years. It has been used to treat fatigue, impotence, insomnia, and high blood pressure, and to regulate blood sugar. Ginseng is available as a powder, paste, in tablets and capsules, and as a tea. People also chew the root; however, it has a bitter taste. Although it has been in use for thousands of years, the medicinal effects of this root haven't adequately been studied by scientific researchers. Therefore we are unable to make recommendations or discuss special needs.

Glutamine: Douglas W. Wilmore, M.D., of Harvard Medical School, says it is "the most common amino acid in the body, a key to the metabolism and maintenance of muscle, the primary energy source for the entire immune system . . . necessary for wound healing and tissue repair. It is also beneficial to those under a great deal of stress."[2] Since this amino acid is widely available in food, no supplements are necessary and we have no special need recommendations.

Glutathione (GSH): This important component of the body's antioxidant defense system is found in plant and animal tissues. It is manufactured by the human body when adequate nutrients, especially glutamine, are available. A generous intake of the antioxidants discussed in this book will assure adequate glutathione in the body. In 1989, researchers from Emory University, using a list of foods compiled by the National Cancer Institute that comprise 90 percent or more of the American diet, measured the GSH content of these foods. Fresh meats, fish, poultry and fresh fruits and vegetables were found to have substantially higher GSH content than canned or processed foods. Good sources of this nutrient are citrus fruits such as oranges and tangerines, and melons such as cantaloupe and watermelons. Vegetables with the most GSH include avocado, asparagus, squash, potato, okra, cauliflower, broccoli, and raw tomatoes. Spinach, carrots, beets, and plain frozen mixed vegetables have moderately high GSH content, according to the Emory researchers.

Recommendation: Eat a wide variety of the antioxidant, phytochemical-rich foods mentioned in this book.

Lycopene: Another form of carotene widely available through diet. Recent research reported that men who eat at least ten servings per week of lycopene-rich, tomato-based foods are 45 percent *less likely* to develop prostate cancer. Like beta-carotene, it is easy to get adequate amounts of this substance just by following normal eating procedures. Supplementation is not needed.

Melatonin: See Chapter 13, "Melatonin Update."

Recommendation: If you have trouble sleeping, try 1 mg or 1.5 mg (one-third to one-half of the 3-mg tablets commonly sold).

Special needs: Individuals flying across many time zones may experience fatigue-producing, concentration-wrecking jet lag. If you do, take one 3-mg tablet on the evening of your arrival. Take either a 1.5- or a 3-mg dose nightly for the next week. Read Chapter 13.

Pycnogenol: These potent antioxidant/phytochemical compounds are extracted from the bark of pine trees or grape seeds. This mixture of phytochemicals is sometimes called proanthocyanidins and sometimes termed oligomeric proanthocyanidins and abbreviated as OPCs or sometimes as PCOs. They have an interesting historical background. During the winter of 1534–35 in what was to become Canada, sailors under the command of French explorer Jacques Cartier were dying of scurvy, which we now know is caused by a deficiency of vitamin C. A Native American from what is now the Quebec area shared information about a healing tea made from pine bark. Cartier had this tea prepared and remarked in his journal about the sailors' dramatic improvement from the symptoms of scurvy. Subsequent studies have documented that the Pycnogenol compounds in pine bark tea are potent antioxidants that "refresh" or extend the capabilities of vitamin C. The content and purity of compounds sold as Pycnogenol may vary.

Recommendation: None.

Special needs: Persons who are concerned about their risk of developing cancer may wish to take 50 mg daily. Individuals diagnosed as having cancer are advised to take 50 mg daily.

Selenium: A mineral with antioxidant properties. Selenium and vitamins C and E are thought to act synergistically (better with each other than individually) to boost immunity and strengthen the cardiovascular system. The recommended dietary allowance (RDA) is 70 mcg for men and 55 mcg for women.

Recommendation: Take a supplement containing at least 60 mcg per day. Selenium should be taken as part of a meal or with some fat to enhance absorption from the intestine.

Special needs: People who want to participate in our tailored protection program (see Table 8.1) or those with heart disease or cancer are advised to take 120 mcg daily.

Tea, black or green: Most people in North America and Europe drink fermented black tea, which accounts for four-fifths of all the tea sold worldwide. People in some Asian countries mostly consume green tea, which is simply unfermented tea made by steaming or drying fresh tea leaves at high temperatures. Recent research indicates that drinking green tea may lower the risk for cancer, especially esophageal cancer. Green tea also reduces high blood pressure and inhibits the clumping of blood platelets, and thus may also protect against heart attack and stroke. While most of the research excitement has been about green tea, a few studies indicate that even black tea may have health-enhancing effects. A study in the July 1, 1994, issue of *Cancer Research* indicates that both black and green teas inhibited skin tumors in lab animals. An earlier study in Sweden found that black-tea drinkers had significantly lower rates of stomach cancer than those who drank beverages other than tea. Both types of tea contain health-promoting substances known as polyphenols, which act as antioxidants; however, unfermented green teas may contain more polyphenols than black teas. Research is needed to confirm this.

Recommendation: Two cups of green tea daily. If you can't get green tea, use any of the black teas. Decaffeinated teas have fewer polyphenols and lower antioxidant effects.

Vitamin C: This water-soluble vitamin carries out its antioxidant functions in the blood and places where water can cross membranes. The RDA is 60 mg for both men and women.

Recommendation: Everyone should take 250 mg of vitamin C twice daily.

Special needs: Smokers or anyone concerned about the health risks addressed in Table 8.1 should take 500 mg twice daily. Vitamin C is the primary antioxidant in the lungs, where this vitamin protects against free radicals. Evidence indicates that vitamin C bolsters antioxidant defenses in the lungs; however, the best health-smart action smokers can take is to become nonsmokers.[3]

Vitamin E: This fat-soluble vitamin does its work inside cells and in intrabody locations where fat can pass through membranes. The RDA is 15 IU for men and 12 IU for women.

Recommendation: 400 IU per day.

Special needs: Individuals concerned about the health risks addressed in Table 8.1 should take 800 IU per day.

Wine, red: Red wine is rich in antioxidant health-promoting substances called polyphenols, which reduce risk for heart disease. Similar polyphenols are in purple grapes and juice from those grapes.

Recommendation: One 6-oz glass of red wine *or* 6 oz of purple grape juice *or* 20 large grapes daily.

Special needs: Men and women with family histories of heart disease should take different amounts. Men should drink two glasses (12 oz total) of wine per day, while women should limit their intake to two small glasses (8 oz). Twelve oz of purple grape juice *or* two servings of purple grapes (40 large grapes) daily can be used by teetotalers.

Zinc: A mineral the human immune system needs to function at peak performance. Deficiency of zinc results in impaired immunocompetence.

Recommendation: 15 mg daily.

APPENDIX B

TABLE B   BETA-CAROTENE AND VITAMIN C CONTENT OF COMMONLY USED VEGETABLES AND FRUITS*

Food	Serving Size	B-carotene, mg	Score	Vitamin C, mg	Score
RDA (Recommended Dietary Allowance)		6 mg	100	60 mg	100
Apple, raw	One	0.03	1	8	13
Apricots, dried	10 halves	6.2	103	1	2
Apricots, fresh	2	2.5	42	8	13
Asparagus	1/2 cup	0.45	8	9	15
Banana	1	0	0	10	17
Beet greens	1/2 cup	2.6	43	23	38
Beets	1/2 cup	0	0	0	0
Broccoli, cooked	1/2 cup	1	17	58	97
Brussels sprouts	1/2 cup	0.48	8	48	80
Cabbage, red, cooked	1/2 cup	0.02	0	26	43
Cantaloupe	1/2	4.8	80	94	157
Carrot juice	1 cup	18	300	16	27
Carrots, raw	1 medium	14.4	240	6	10
Cauliflower, cooked	1/2 cup	0.01	0	28	47
Celery, raw	1/2 cup	0.42	7	5	8
Corn, yellow	1/2 cup	0.05	1	5	8
Cranberries, raw	1/2 cup	0.002	0	100	167
Cucumber, raw	1/2 cup	0.006	0	2	3
Currants, black	1/4 cup	0.06	1	51	85
Eggplant, raw	1/2 cup	0.04	1	1	2
Gazpacho	1 cup	11.7	195	3	5
Grapefruit, pink	1/2	1.6	27	47	78

Food	Serving Size	B-carotene, mg	Score	Vitamin C, mg	Score
Grapefruit, white	1/2	0.001	0	83	138
Grapefruit juice, pink	6 fl oz	0.8	13	70	117
Grapes, raw	12	0.02	0	5	8
Green beans	1/2 cup	0.35	6	6	10
Greens, turnip, cooked	1/2 cup	3.9	65	20	33
Kale, cooked	1/2 cup	3	50	27	45
Kiwi	1	0.04	2.6	75	125
Lettuce, romaine	1 cup	1.1	18	18	30
Mango	1/2	1.4	23	29	48
Nectarine, raw	1	0.1	2	7	12
Onion, yellow, raw	1/2 cup	0.08	1	5	8
Oranges, California, navel	1	0.04	1	80	133
Oranges, Florida	1	0.04	1	68	113
Orange juice	6 fl oz	0.01	0	93	155
Peaches, raw	1 medium	0.1	2	6	10
Pears, raw	1 medium	0.02	0	6	10
Peas, green	1/2 cup	0.3	5	11	18
Peppers, sweet, green, raw	1/2 cup	0.14	2	45	75
Peppers, sweet, red, raw	1/2 cup	1.4	23	95	158
Peppers, hot, raw	1/4 cup	0.7	12	91	152
Pineapple, canned	1/2 cup	0.02	0	0	0
Potato, baked with skin	1 large	0	0	26	43
Pumpkin, cooked	1/2 cup	3.7	62	4	7
Radish, raw	1/2 cup	0.004	0	13	22
Snow peas with pod	1/2 cup	0.03	1	38	63
Spinach, cooked	1/2 cup	4.9	82	25	42
Squash, summer, cooked	1/2 cup	0.4	7	0	0
Squash, winter, cooked	1/2 cup	2.9	48	13	22
Strawberries, raw	1/2 cup	0.009	0	41	68
Sweet potatoes, cooked	1/2 medium	6.6	110	28	47
Tangerine, raw	1 large	0.04	1	26	43

Food	Serving Size	B-carotene, mg	Score	Vitamin C, mg	Score
Tomato, raw	1 medium	0.62	10	34	57
Tomato juice	6 fl oz	1.5	25	34	57
Vegetable juice	6 fl oz	2	40	36	60
Vegetable soup	1 cup	1.9	32	3	5
Watermelon, raw	1 cup	0.37	6	46	77

* This information has been collected from many sources including published articles and manufacturers.

**Score is percentage of recommended dietary allowance.

NOTES

CHAPTER 1

1. William A. Pryor, "Measurement of Oxidative Stress Status in Humans," *Cancer Epidemiology, Biomarkers,* Vol. 7 (May–June 1993), and *Prevention,* Vol. 2, May/June 1993), p. 289.
2. Natalie Angier, "Free Radicals: The Price We Pay for Breathing," *The New York Times Magazine* (April 25, 1993), p. 62.
3. John M. Gutteridge, "Antioxidants, Nutritional Supplements, and Life-Threatening diseases," *British Journal of Biomedical Science,* Vol. 31 (1994), pp. 288–95.
4. Bruce N. Ames et al., "Oxidants, Antioxidants, and the Degenerative Diseases of Aging," *Proceedings of the National Academy of Science,* Vol. 90 (September 1993), pp. 7915–22.

CHAPTER 2

1. To protect privacy, Martin and Suzanne are composite characters. They don't exist exactly as they are described but they are based on real individuals. There are many Martins and Suzannes in our world.
2. Denham Harman, "Free Radical Theory of Aging: History," pp. 1–11; V. K. Koltover, "Free Radical Theory of Aging: View Against the Reliability Theory," pp. 11–20; and M. G. Simic, "The Rate of DNA Damage and Aging, pp. 20–31, in *Free Radicals and Aging,* (ed.) Ingrid Emerit and Britton Chance (Stuttgart: Birkhäuser Verlag, 1992). Also, James E. Engstrom et al. found that "Standard mortality rates for persons with the highest vitamin C intake" have substantially reduced risks from deaths "for all causes and all cardiovascular diseases among males, females, and both sexes combined." In "Vitamin C Intake and Mortality Among a Sample of the United States Population," *Epidemiology,* Vol. 3, No. 2 (May 1992), p. 197.
3. Trudy R. Turner and Mark L. Weiss, "The Genetics of Longevity in Humans," *Biological Anthropology and Aging: Perspectives on Human*

Variation Over the Life Span, ed. D. E. Crews and R. M. Garruto (New York: Oxford University Press, 1994), pp. 76–100.

4. Eva P. Shronts, "11 Basic Concepts of Immunology and Its Application to Clinical Nutrition," *Nutrition in Clinical Practice,* #4, (1993), p. 177; also *Lancet,* Vol. 340 (November 7, 1992), pp. 1124–27.

5. Samuel Goldstein, "The Biology of Aging: Looking to Defuse the Genetic Time Bomb," *Geriatrics,* Vol. 48, No. 9 (September 1993), pp. 75–82.

6. Leonard Hayflick, "Aging Under Glass," *How and Why We Age* (New York: Ballantine Books, 1994), pp. 111–36.

7. James F. Scheer, "Vitamin E: Our Prime Protectant," *Better Nutrition for Today's Living,* Vol. 56 (October 1994), p. 46.

8. Denham Harman, "Free-Radical Theory of Aging: Increasing Functional Life Span," *Pharmacology of Aging Processes: Methods of Assessment and Potential Interventions* in *Annals of the New York Academy of Sciences,* Vol. 717 (June 30, 1994), p. 1.

9. J. B. Blumberg, "Interactions Between Vitamin E, Free Radicals, and Immunity During the Aging Process, in *Free Radicals in Diagnostic Medicine,* ed. D. Armstrong (New York: Plenum, 1994), p. 325.

10. Rebecca Voelker, "Radical Approaches: Is Widespread Testing and Treatment for Oxidative Injuries Coming Soon?" *JAMA,* Vol. 270, No. 17 (November 3, 1993), p. 2024.

11. W. A. Pryor, "The Free Radical Theory of Aging Revisited: A Critique and a Suggested Disease-Specific Theory," in *Modern Biological Theories of Aging,* Vol. 31, ed. Huber R. Warner et al. (New York: Raven Press, 1987). p. 234

12. J. Steven Richardson, "Free Radicals and Alzheimer's Disease," *Proceedings of the Alzheimer's Association Annual Meeting, Research Update Session.* (October, 1992), p. 13.

13. Natalie Angier, "Free Radicals: The Price We Pay for Breathing," *The New York Times Magazine* (April 25, 1993), p. 62.

14. Anthony T. Diplock, "Antioxidant Nutrients and Disease Prevention: An Overview," *American Journal of Clinical Nutrition,* Vol. 53 (1991), p. 189S.

15. Z. Zaman et al., "Plasma Concentrations of Vitamins A and E and Carotenoids in Alzheimer's Disease," *Age and Ageing,* Vol. 21 (1992), pp. 91–94.

16. Denham Harman, "Free-Radical Theory of Aging: Increasing the Functional Life Span," *Pharmacology of Aging Processes: Methods of Assessment and Potential Interventions* in *Annals of the New York Academy of Sciences,* Vol. 717 (June 30, 1994), p. 5.

17. John and Ann Carney, "Role of Protein Oxidation in Aging and in Age-

Associated Neurodegenerative Diseases," *Life Science,* Vol. 55, No. 25–26 (1994), pp. 1–7.

18. Charles D. Smith, John M. Carney, Tohru Tatsumo, et al., "Protein Oxidation in Aging Brain," *Annals of the New York Academy of Sciences: Aging and Cellular Defense Mechanism,* Vol. 663 (1993), pp. 110–19.

19. Richardson, "Free Radicals and Alzheimer's Disease."

20. M. J. Stampfer et al., "Vitamin E Consumption and the Risk of Coronary Disease in Women," *New England Journal of Medicine,* Vol. 328 (May 20, 1993), pp. 1444–49.

21. Eric B. Rimm et al., "Vitamin E Consumption and Risk of Coronary Disease in Men," *New England Journal of Medicine,* Vol. 328 (May 20, 1993), pp. 1450–56.

22. Gladys Block, "Dietary Guidelines and the Results of Food Consumption Servings," *American Journal of Clinical Nutrition,* Vol. 53 (1991), p. 356S.

23. Ranjit K. Chandra, "Effect of Vitamin and Trace-Element Supplementation on Immune Responses and Infection in Elderly Subjects," *Lancet,* Vol. 340 (1992), pp. 1124–27.

24. Breecher interview with Dr. Blumberg. Also "Vitamins, Trace Elements, and Immunologic Youth?", *Patient Care* (March 16, 1993), pp. 21–22.

25. Chandra, "Effect of Vitamin and Trace-Element Supplementation."

26. Breecher interview with Meydani et al., "Antioxidants and the Aging Immune Response," in *Antioxidants, Nutrients, and Immune Functions,* ed. Adrianne Bendich, Marshall Phillips, and Robert P. Tengerdy (New York: Plenum, 1988), p. 57.

27. John Bogden, et al., "Daily Micronutrient Supplements Enhance Delayed Hypersensitivity Skin Test Results in Older People," *American Journal of Clinical Nutrition,* Vol. 60, No. 3 (September 1994), p. 437.

28. Anthony T. Diplock, "Antioxidant Nutrients and Disease," *Nutrition and Health,* Vol. 9 (1993), pp. 37–42; N. D. Penn et al., "The Effect of Dietary Supplementation with Vitamins A, C, and E on Cell-Mediated Immune Function in Elderly Long-Stay Patients: A Randomized Controlled Trial," *Age and Ageing,* Vol. 20 (1991), pp. 169–74.

29. Kenneth H. Cooper, M.D., *Dr. Kenneth H. Cooper's Antioxidant Revolution* (Nashville: Thomas Nelson, 1994), p. 119.

CHAPTER 3

1. R. W. Alexander, "Inflammation and Coronary Heart Disease," *The New England Journal of Medicine,* Vol. 331 (1994), pp. 468–69.
2. D. Steinberg, "Clinical Trials of Antioxidants in Atherosclerosis: Are We Doing the Right Thing?" *Lancet,* Vol. 346 (1995), pp. 36–38.
3. J. Regnstrom, J. Nilsson, P. Tornvall, C. Landou, and A. Hamsten, "Susceptibility to Low-Density Lipoprotein Oxidation and Coronary Atherosclerosis in Man," *Lancet,* Vol. 339 (1992), pp. 1183–86.
4. K. F. Gey, "Inverse Correlation Between Plasma Vitamin E and Mortality from Ischemic Heart Disease in Cross-Cultural Epidemiology," *American Journal of Clinical Nutrition,* Vol. 53 (1991), pp. 326S–34S.
5. R. A. Riemersma, D. A. Wood, C. C. A. Macintyre, R. A. Elton, K. F. Gey, and M. F. Oliver, "Risk of Angina Pectoris and Plasma Concentrations of Vitamins A, C, and E and Carotene," *Lancet,* Vol. 337 (1991), pp. 1–5.
6. E. B. Rimm, M. J. Stampfer, A. Ascherio, E. Giovannucci, G. A. Colditz, and W. Willett, "Vitamin E Consumption and the Risk of Coronary Heart Disease in Men," *The New England Journal of Medicine,* Vol. 328 (1993), pp. 1450–56.
7. M. J. Stampfer, C. H. Hennekens, J. E. Manson, G. A. Colditz, B. Rosner, and W. C. Willett, "Vitamin E Consumption and the Risk of Coronary Disease in Women," *The New England Journal of Medicine,* Vol. 328 (1993), pp. 1444–49.
8. A. F. M. Kardinaal, F. J. Kok, J. Ringstad, J. Gomez-Aracena, V. P. Mazaev, L. Kohlmeier, et al., "Antioxidants in Adipose Tissue and Risk of Myocardial Infarction: The EURAMIC Study," *Lancet,* Vol. 342 (1993), pp. 1379–84.
9. J. M. Gaziano, "Antioxidant Vitamins and Coronary Artery Disease Risk," *American Journal of Medicine,* Vol. 97 (Suppl. 3A) (1994), pp. 19S–21S.
10. J. M. Gaziano, J. E. Manson, L. G. Branch, F. LaMott, J. E. Colditz, and C. H. Hennekens, "Dietary Beta-carotene Intake and Decreased Cardiovascular Mortality in an Elderly Cohort," *Journal of the American College of Cardiology,* Vol. 19 (1992), p. 377.
11. D. L. Morris, S. B. Kritchevsky, and C. E. Davis, "Serum Caretenoids and Coronary Heart Disease: The Lipid Research Clinic Coronary Primary Prevention Trial and Follow-up Study," *JAMA,* Vol. 272 (1994), pp. 1439–41.

12. D. A. Street, G. W. Comstock, R. M. Salkeld, W. Schuep, and M. J. Klag, "Serum Antioxidants and Myocardial Infarction: Are Low Levels of Carotenoids and Alpha-tocopherol Risk Factors for Myocardial Infarction?" *Circulation,* Vol. 90 (1994), pp. 1154–61.

13. J. E. Enstrom, L. E. Kanim, and M. A. Klein, "Vitamin C Intake and a Sample of the United States Population," *American Journal of Epidemiology,* Vol. 3 (1992), pp. 194–202.

14. M. G. L. Hertog, E. J. M. Feskens, P. C. H. Hollman, M. B. Katan, and D. Kromhout, "Dietary Antioxidant Flavonoids and Risk of Coronary Heart Disease: The Zutphen Elderly Study," *Lancet,* Vol. 342 (1993), pp. 1107–11.

15. B. Fuhrman, A. Lavy, and M. Aviram, "Consumption of Red Wine with Meals Reduces the Susceptibility of Human Plasma and Low-Density Lipoprotein to Lipid Peroxidation, *American Journal of Clinical Nutrition,* Vol. 61 (1995), pp. 549–54.

16. M. J. Stampfer, and M. R. Malinow, "Can Lowering Homocysteine Levels Reduce Cardiovascular Risk?" *The New England Journal of Medicine,* Vol. 332 (1995), pp. 328–29.

17. J. B. Ubbink, W. J. Vermaak, A. van der Merwe, and P. J. Becker, "Vitamin B_{12}, Vitamin B_6, and Folate Nutritional Status in Men with Hyperhomocysteinemia," *American Journal of Clinical Nutrition,* Vol. 57 (1993), pp. 47–53.

18. J. W. Anderson and N. J. Gustafson, *Dr. Anderson's High Fiber Fitness Plan,* (Lexington: University Press of Kentucky, 1994), pp. 1–250.

CHAPTER 4

1. W. J. Blot, J.-Y. Li, P. R. Taylor, W. Guo, S. Dawsey, G.-Q. Wang, et al., "Nutrition Intervention Trials in Linxian, China: Supplementation with Specific Vitamin/Mineral Combinations, Cancer Incidence, and Disease-Specific Mortality in the General Population," *Journal of the National Cancer Institute,* Vol. 85 (1993), pp. 1483–92.

2. W. J. Blot, J. Li, P. R. Taylor, and B. Li, "Lung Cancer and Vitamin Supplementation," *The New England Journal of Medicine,* Vol. 331 (1994), p. 614.

3. T. Beardsley, "A War Not Won," *Scientific American,* Vol. 270, No. 1, (1994), pp. 130–38.

4. National Academy of Sciences, *Diet and Health* (Washington, DC: National Academy Press, 1989), p. 1.

5. T. Byers and G. Perry, "Dietary Carotenes, Vitamin C, and Vitamin E as

Protective Antioxidants in Human Cancers," *Annual Review of Nutrition,* Vol. 12 (1992), pp. 139–59.

6. P. A. Lachance, "Micronutrients in Cancer Prevention," in *Food Phytochemicals for Cancer Prevention,* ed. M.-T. Huang, T. Osawa, C.-T. Ho, and R. T. Rosen (Washington, DC: American Chemical Society, 1994), pp. 49–64.

7. L. Kohlmeier, "Epidemiology of Anticarcinogens in Food," in *Nutrition and Biotechnology in Heart Disease and Cancer,* ed. J. B. Longenecker et al. (New York: Plenum, 1995), pp. 125–39.

8. H. Gerster, "Beta-carotene, Vitamin E, and Vitamin C in Different Stages of Experimental Carcinogenesis," *European Journal of Clinical Nutrition,* Vol. 49 (1995), pp. 155–68.

9. T. J. Slaga, "Inhibition of the Induction of Cancer by Antioxidants," in Longenecker et al., eds., *Nutrition and Biotechnology in Heart Disease and Cancer,* pp. 167–74.

10. B. G. Sanders and K. Kline, "Nutrition, Immunology, and Cancer: An Overview," in Longenecker et al., eds., *Nutrition and Biotechnology in Heart Disease and Cancer,* pp. 185–94.

11. D. Schardt, "Phytochemicals: Plants Against Cancer," *Nutrition Action Health Letter,* Vol. 21 (1994), pp. 8–11.

12. Y. H. He and C. Kies, "Green and Black Tea Consumption in Humans: Impact on Polyphenol Concentrations in Feces, Blood, and Urine," *Plant Food and Human Nutrition,* Vol. 46 (1994), pp. 221–29.

13. K. A. Steinmetz and J. D. Potter, "Vegetables, Fruit, and Cancer: Epidemiology," *Cancer Causes & Control,* Vol. 2 (1991), pp. 325–57.

14. G. Block, B. Patterson, and A. Subar, "Fruits, Vegetables, and Cancer Prevention: A Review of the Epidemiologic Evidence," *Nutrition and Cancer,* Vol. 18 (1992), pp. 1–29.

15. R. Zeigler, "Vegetables, Fruits, and Carotenoids and the Risk of Cancer," *American Journal of Clinical Nutrition,* Vol. 53 (1991), pp. 251S–259S.

16. J. Weisburger, "Nutritional Approach to Cancer Prevention with Emphasis on Vitamins, Antioxidants, and Carotenoids," *American Journal of Clinical Nutrition,* Vol. 53 (1991), pp. 226S–237S.

17. K. A. Steinmetz and J. D. Potter, "Vegetables, Fruit, and Cancer: II, Mechanisms," *Cancer Causes and Control,* Vol. 2 (1991), pp. 427–42.

18. S. T. Mayne, D. T. Janerich, P. Greenwald, S. Chorost, K. Tucci, B. Zaman, et al., "Dietary Beta-carotene and Lung Cancer Risk in U.S. Nonsmokers," *Journal of the National Cancer Institute,* Vol. 86 (1994), pp. 33–38.

19. M. Messina, V. Messina, and K. Setchell, *The Simple Soybean and Your Health,* (Garden City Park, NY: Avery, 1994).

20. M. J. Messina, V. Persky, K. D. B. Setchell and S. Barnes, "Soy Intake and Cancer Risk: A Review of the in Vitro and in Vivo Data," *Nutrition and Cancer,* Vol. 21 (1994), pp. 113–31.

21. D. Zaridze, V. Filipchenko, V. Kustov, V. Serdyuk, and S. Duffy, "Diet and Colorectal Cancer: Results of Two Case-Control Studies in Russia," *European Journal of Cancer,* Vol. 29A (1993), pp. 112–15.

22. The Alpha-Tocopherol BC: The Effect of Vitamin E and Beta-carotene on the Incidence of Lung Cancer and Other Cancers in Male Smokers," *The New England Journal of Medicine,* Vol. 330 (1994), pp. 1029–34.

23. E. W. Flagg, R. J. Coates, and R. S. Greenberg, "Epidemiologic Studies of Antioxidants and Cancer in Humans," *Journal of the American College of Nutrition,* Vol. 14 (1995), pp. 419–27.

24. Council for Responsible Nutrition, *Scientists Support Health Claims for Antioxidant Vitamins* (Washington, DC: Council for Responsible Nutrition, 1992), p. 1.

25. E. B. Rimm, M. J. Stampfer, A. Ascherio, E. Giovannucci, G. A. Colditz, and W. Willett, "Vitamin E Consumption and the Risk of Coronary Heart Disease in Men," *The New England Journal of Medicine,* Vol. 328 (1993), pp. 1450–56.

26. M. J. Stampfer, C. H. Hennekens, J. E. Manson, G. A. Colditz, B. Rosner, and W. C. Willett, "Vitamin E Consumption and the Risk of Coronary Disease in Women," *The New England Journal of Medicine,* Vol. 328 (1993), pp. 1444–49.

27. R. K. Boutwell, "Nutrition and Carcinogenesis: Historical Highlights and Future Prospects," in Longenecker, et al., eds., *Nutrition and Biotechnology in Heart Disease and Cancer,* pp. 111–23.

CHAPTER 5

1. L. Frolich and P. Riederer, "Free Radical Mechanisms in Dementia of Alzheimer Type and the Potential for Antioxidative Treatment," *Drug Research,* Vol. 45, No. 1 (1995), pp. 443–46.

2. John M. Carney and Ann M. Carney, and D. A. Butterfield. "Aging."

3. R. J. Reiter, "Oxidative Processes and Antioxidant Mechanisms in the Aging Brain," *FASEB Journal* (1995), p. 526.

4. J. Steven Richardson, "Free Radicals and Alzheimer's Disease," *In Search of Treatment for Alzheimer's Disease: The Role of Basic Research.* (Chicago: The Alzheimer's Association, 1993), pp. 10–14.

5. Richard P. White and James T. Robertson, "Basic Concepts of Antioxidant Therapy," *Journal of the Tennessee Medical Association,* Vol. 88, No. 2 (1995), pp. 54–58.

236

6. P. H. Evans, et al., "Oxidative Damage in Alzheimer's Dementia, and the Potential Etiopathogenic Role of Aluminosilicates, Microglia, and Micronutrient Interactions," in *Free Radicals and Aging*, ed. I. Emerit and B. Chance. (Basel: Bukhäuser Verlag, 1992), pp. 178–89.

7. David A. Bennett and Denis A. Evans, "Alzheimer's Disease: Epidemiology and Public Health Impact," *Disease-a-Month*, Vol. 37, No. 1 (1992), p. 13.

8. Evans, "Oxidative Damage in Alzheimer's Dementia," p. 178.

9. Richardson, "Free Radicals and Alzheimer's Disease," p. 13.

10. D. J. Selkoe, "Amyloid Protein and Alzheimer's Disease," *Scientific American*, Vol. 265, No. 5 (1991), pp. 68–78.

11. Ibid.

12. Frolich and Riederer, "Free Radical Mechanisms," *Drug Research*, p. 445.

13. Evans, "Oxidative Damage in Alzheimer's Dementia," p. 184.

14. T. Yoshikawa, "Free Radicals and Their Scavengers in Parkinson's Disease," *Journal of European Neurology*, Vol. 33, Supp. 1 (1993), pp. 60–68.

15. Bennett and Evans, "Alzheimer's Disease," p. 32.

16. Frolich and Riederer, "Free Radical Mechanisms," *Drug Research*, p. 444.

17. Mohsen Meydani, "Vitamin E Requirements in Relation to Dietary Fish Oil and Oxidative Stress in the Elderly," in *Free Radicals and Aging*, ed. I. Emerit and B. Chance, Zurich, Switzerland, Bukhäuser Verlag, 1992 p. 411–418.

18. Stanley Fahn, *Annals of Neurology*, Vol. 32 (1992), pp. S128–S32. Also Yoshikawa, "Free Radicals and Their Scavengers," p. 66.

19. Fahn, *Annals of Neurology*, pp. S128–132.

20. Y. Stern et al., "Influence of Education and Occupation on the Incidence of Alzheimer's Disease," *JAMA*, Vol. 271, No. 13 (1994), pp. 1004–10.

21. Daniel Golden, "Building a Better Brain," *Life* (July 1994), p. 65.

22. Miriam Ehrenberg and Otto Ehrenberg, *Optimum Brain Power: A Total Program for Increasing Your Intelligence* (New York: Dodd, Mead, 1987).

23. The authors acknowledge the aid given this section by Drs. Marian and Otto Ehrenberg in interviews with coauthor Breecher in the past. We recommend their book cited above. We also tip our hats to Harold H. Bloomfield, M.D., and Robert K. Cooper, Ph.D., authors of *The Power of 5*. Dr. Bloomfield's expertise has been utilized several times over the years in interviews by coauthor Breecher. *The Power of 5* published by Rodale Press in 1995 is a book we recommend.

24. Raymond Harris, *Fitness After 50.*
25. Coauthor Breecher interviewed Dr. Harris on this subject. Among the many studies that support this statement are the following:

- Robert L. Rogers, et al., "After Reaching Retirement Age Physical Activity Sustains Cerebral Perfusion and Cognition," *Journal of the American Geriatrics Society,* Vol. 38 (1990), pp. 123–28.
- L. Clarkson-Smith and A. A. Hartley, "Relationships Between Physical Exercise and Cognitive Abilities in Older Adults," *Psychology and Aging,* Vol. 41, No. 2 (1989), pp. 183–89.
- W. E. Sime, "Psychological Benefits of Exercise," *Advances,* Vol. 1, No. 4 (1984), pp. 15–29.
- A. H. Ismail and Abdel El-Naggar, "Effect of Exercise on Cognitive Processing in Adult Men," *The Journal of Human Ergology,* Vol. 10, No. 1 (1981), pp. 83–91.
- Waneen Wyrick Spirduso, "Physical Fitness, Aging, and Psychomotor Speed: A Review," *Journal of Gerontology,* Vol. 35, No. 6 (1980), pp. 850–65.

CHAPTER 6

1. Joseph P. Bark, *Your Skin . . . An Owner's Guide* (Englewood Cliffs, NJ: Prentice Hall, 1995), p. 2.
2. Vitamin E Research and Information Service (VERIS), "Vitamin E Research Summary: The Role of Vitamin E in Skin Care and Protection" (1994).
3. Ingrid Emerit, "Free Radicals and Aging of the Skin," in *Free Radicals and Aging,* ed. Ingrid Emerit and Britton Chance, (Basel: Birkhäuser Verlag, 1992), pp. 333, 337.
4. Emerit, "Free Radicals," p. 339.
5. Unless otherwise noted, the following information has been compiled from educational materials published by the Arthritis Foundation and the National Institute of Arthritis, Musculoskeletal and Skin Diseases or from interviews with their representatives.
6. Y. Henrotin et al., "Active Oxygen Species, Articular Inflammation, and Cartilage Damage," in Emerit and Chance, eds., *Free Radicals and Aging,* p. 315.
7. Ibid., p. 316.
8. K. H. Schmidt and W. Bayer, "Efficacy of Vitamin E as a Drug in Inflammatory Joint Disease," in *Antioxidants in Therapy and Preventative Medicine,* ed. I. Emerit et al. (New York: Plenum, 1990), pp. 147–50.

238

9. Henrotin, "Active Oxygen Species," pp. 317–18.

10. Guilherme P. Deucher, "Antioxidant Therapy in the Aging Process," in Emerit and Chance, eds., *Free Radicals and Aging,* p. 428.

11. Paul E. Jennings, "From Hemobiology to Vasculaer Disease: A Review of the Potential of Gliclazide to Influence the Pathogenesis of Diabetic Vascular Disease," *Journal of Diabetes and Its Complications,* Vol. 84, No. 4 (1994), pp. 226–30.

12. J. Ludvigsson, "Intervention at Diagnosis of Type I Diabetes Using Either Antioxidants or Photopheresis," *Diabetes-Metablolism Reviews,* Vol. 9, No. 4 (1993), pp. 329–36.

13. J. W. Anderson, *Professional Guide to High Fiber Fitness Plan* (Lexington, KY HCF Nutrition Foundation, 1995).

14. J. W. Anderson, *Diabetes: A Practical New Guide to Healthy Living* (1981).

15. S. P. Helmrich, D. R. Ragland, R. W. Lueng, and R. S. Paffenbarger, "Physical Activity and Reduced Occurrence of Non-Insulin-Dependent Diabetes Mellitus," *The New England Journal of Medicine,* Vol. 325 (1991), pp. 147–52.

16. The terms "glucose" and "sugar" are used interchangeably here.

17. Marie McCarren, "Intensive Therapy Reduces the Risk of Diabetic Eye, Kidney, and Nerve Disease," *Diabetic Forecast,* Vol. 46, No. 9 (1993), pp. 28–51.

18. C. J. Dillard, K. J. Kunert, and A. L. Tappel, "Effects of Vitamin E, Ascorbic Acid, and Mannitol on Alloxan-Induced Lipid Peroxidation in Rats," *Archives of Biochemical Biophysics,* Vol. 216 (1982), pp. 204–12.

19. J. V. Hunt, R. T. Dean, and S. P. Wolff, "Hydroxyl Radical Production and Autoxidative Glycosylation," *Biochemistry Journal,* Vol. 256 (1988), pp. 205–12.

20. A. Szczeklik, R. J. Gryglewski, B. Domagala, R. Dworski, and R. Basista, "Dietary Supplementation with Vitamin E in Hyperlipoproteinemias: Effects on Plasma Lipid Peroxides, Antioxidant Activity, Prostacyclin Generation, and Platelet Aggregation," *Thrombosis Haemostasis,* Vol. 54 (1985), pp. 425–30.

21. A. Ceriello, A. Quatraro, and D. Guigliano, "New Insights on Nonenzymatic Glycosylation May Lead to Therapeutic Approaches for the Prevention of Diabetic Complications," *Diabetic Medicine,* Vol. 9 (1992), pp. 297–99.

22. James W. Anderson et al., "Postprandial Serum Glucose, Insulin, and Lipoprotein Responses to High- and Low-Fiber Diets," *Metabolism,* Vol. 44, No. 7 (1995), pp. 848–54.

23. James W. Anderson, Belinda M. Smith, and Nancy J. Gustafson, "Health Benefits and Practical Aspects of High-Fiber Diets," *American Journal of Clinical Nutrition*, Vol. 59, No. 5 (1994), pp. 1242S–47S. James W. Anderson et al., "Metabolic Effects of High-Carbohydrate, High-Fiber Diets for Insulin-Dependent Diabetic Individuals," *American Journal of Clinical Nutrition*, Vol. 54 (1991), pp. 936–43.

24. M. J. Franz et al., "Nutrition Recommendations and Principles for People with Diabetes Mellitus," *Diabetes Care*, Vol. 17, No. 5 (1994), pp. 519–22.

25. National Advisory Eye Council, *Vision Research a National Plan, 1994–1998*. National Institutes of Health Publication 93-3186. 1994. Washington, DC.

26. G. E. Bunce, "Antioxidant Nutrition and Cataract in Women: A Prospective Study," *Nutrition Reviews*, Vol. 51, No. 3 (1993), pp. 84–85.

27. Johanna M. Seddon, et al., "The Use of Vitamin Supplements and the Risk of Cataract Among U.S. Male Physicians," *American Journal of Public Health*, Vol. 84, No. 5 (1994), pp. 788–92.

28. William G. Christen, "Antioxidants and Eye Disease," *The American Journal of Medicine*, Vol. 97, Supp. 3A (1994), pp. 14S–17S.

29. Davi-Ellen Chabner, *The Language of Medicine* (Philadelphia: W. B. Saunders, 1981), p. 458.

30. James Collins, *Your Eyes . . . An Owner's Guide* (Englewood Cliffs, NJ: Prentice Hall, 1995), p. 149.

31. Stuart P. Richer, "Is There a Prevention and Treatment Strategy for Macular Degeneration?" *Journal of the American Optometric Association*, Vol. 64 (1993), p. 838.

32. Anita M. Van Der Hagen et al., "Free Radicals and Antioxidant Supplementation: A Review of Their Roles in Age-Related Macular Degeneration," *Journal of the American Optometric Association*, Vol. 64 (1993), pp. 871–78.

33. Christen, "Antioxidants and Eye Diseases," pp. 14S–17S.

34. James McD. Robertson et al., "A Possible Role for Vitamins C and E in Cataract Prevention," *American Journal of Clinical Nutrition*, Vol. 53 (1991), pp. 346S–351S.

35. Paul F. Jacques et al., "Antioxidant Status in Persons with and without Senile Cataract," *Archives of Ophthalmology*, Vol. 106 (1988), pp. 337–40.

36. J. M. Seddon, "Dietary Carotenoids, Vitamins A, C, and E, and Advanced Age-Related Macular Degeneration," *JAMA*, Vol. 272, No. 18 (1994), pp. 1413–20.

37. Christen, "Antioxidants and Eye Disease," p. 15S.
38. Seddon et al., "The Use of Vitamin Supplements."
39. Kaminski interview by Charlotte Rancillio. Kaminski also was listed as a coauthor in Van Der Hagen et al., "Free Radicals and Antioxidant Supplementation," and used exact language from that article.

CHAPTER 7

1. M. Messina, V. Messina, and K. Setchell, *The Simple Soybean and Your Health* (Garden City Park, NY: Avery, 1994).
2. J. W. Anderson, B. M. Johnstone, and M. E. Cook-Newell, "Meta-analysis of Effects of Soy Protein Intake on Serum Lipids in Humans," *The New England Journal of Medicine,* Vol. 333 (1995), pp. 276–82.
3. M. J. Messina, V. Persky, K. D. R. Setchell, and S. Barnes, "Soy Intake and Cancer Risk: A Review of the in Vitro and in Vivo Data," *Nutrition and Cancer,* Vol. 21 (1994), pp. 113–31.
4. S. Barnes and C. Grubbs, "Soybeans Inhibit Mammary Tumor Growth in Models of Breast Cancer" in *Mutagens and Carcinogens in the Diet,* ed. M. W. Pariza. (New York: Wiley-Liss, 1990), pp. 239–53.
5. J. J. Anderson, W. W. Ambrose, and S. C. Garner, "Orally Dosed Genistein from Soy and Prevention of Cancellous Bone Loss in Two Ovariectomized Rat Models," *Journal of Nutrition,* Vol. 125 (1995), p. 799S.
6. A. Cassidy, S. Bingham, and K. D. R. Setchell, "Biological Effects of a Diet of Soy Protein Rich in Isoflavones on the Menstrual Cycle of Premenopausal Women," *American Journal of Clinical Nutrition,* Vol. 60 (1995), pp. 333–40.
7. A. Chait, J. D. Brunzell, M. A. Denke, D. Eisenberg, N. D. Ernst, F. A. Franklin, Jr., et al., "Rationale of the Diet-Heart Statement of the American Heart Association: Report of the Nutrition Committee." *Circulation,* Vol. 88 (1993), pp. 3008–29.
8. J. E. Manson, H. Tosteson, P. M. Ridker, S. Satterfield, P. Hebert, and G. T. O'Connor, "The Primary Prevention of Myocardial Infarction," *The New England Journal of Medicine,* Vol. 326 (1992), pp. 1406–16.
9. M. S. Anthony, G. L. Burke, C. L. Hughes, and T. B. Clarkson, "Does Soy Supplementation Improve Coronary Heart Disease (CHD) Risk?" *Circulation,* Vol. 91 (1995), p. 925.

CHAPTER 8

1. W. Pierpaoli, W. Regelson, and C. Colman, *The Melatonin Miracle: Nature's Age-Reversing, Disease-Fighting, Sex-Enhancing Hormone* (New York: Simon & Schuster, 1995).
2. R. J. Reiter, D. Tan, B. Poeggeler, A. Menendez-Pelaez, L. Chen, and S. Saarela, "Melatonin as a Free Radical Scavenger: Implications for Aging and Age-Related Diseases," *Annals of the New York Academy of Sciences,* Vol. 719 (1994), pp. 1–12.
3. F. Waldhauser, B. Ehrhart, and E. Forster, "Clinical Aspects of the Melatonin Action: Impact of Development, Aging, and Puberty, Involvement of Melatonin in Psychiatric Disease, and Importance of Neuroimmunoendocrine Interactions," *Experientia,* Vol. 49 (1993), pp. 671–81.
4. R. J. Reiter and J. Robinson, *Melatonin: Your Body's Natural Wonder Drug* (New York: Bantam, 1995).
5. S. M. Armstrong and J. R. Redman, "Melatonin: A Chronobiotic with Antiaging Properties?" *Medical Hypothesis,* Vol. 34 (1991), pp. 300–309.
6. R. A. Passwater and C. Kandaswami, *Pycnogenol: The Super "Protector" Nutrient* (New Canaan, CT: Keats, 1994).
7. J. W. Anderson, *Professional Guide to High-Fiber Fitness Plan* (Lexington, KY: HCF Nutrition Foundation, 1995), pp. 1–13, 24.
8. J. W. Anderson and N. J. Gustafson, *Dr. Anderson's High-Fiber Fitness Plan* (Lexington: University Press of Kentucky, 1994).

CHAPTER 10

1. C. Meyers, *Walking: A Complete Guide to the Complete Exercise* (New York: Random House, 1992).
2. E. B. Larson and R. A. Bruce, "Exercise and Aging," *Annals of Internal Medicine,* Vol. 105 (1986), pp. 783–85.
3. S. N. Blair, H. W. Kohl, N. F. Gordon, and R. S. Paffenbarger, "How Much Physical Activity Is Good for Health?" *Annual Review of Public Health,* Vol. 13 (1992), pp. 99–126.
4. J. W. Anderson, *Professional Guide to High-Fiber Fitness Plan,* (Lexington, KY: HCF Nutrition Foundation, 1995).
5. L. Sandvik, J. Erikssen, G. Erikssen, R. Mundal, and K. Ridahl, "Phys-

ical Fitness as a Predictor of Mortality Among Healthy, Middle-Aged Norwegian Men," *The New England Journal of Medicine,* Vol. 328 (1993), pp. 533–37.

6. R. S. Paffenbarger, R. T. Hyde, A. L. Wing, I.-M. Lee, D. L. Jung, and J. B. Kampert, "The Association of Changes in Physical-Activity Level and Other Lifestyle Characteristics with Mortality Among Men," *The New England Journal of Medicine,* Vol. 328 (1993), pp. 538–45.

7. R. S. Paffenbarger, R. T. Hyde, A. L. Wing, and C.-C. Hsieh, "Physical Activity, All-Cause Mortality, and Longevity of College Alumni," *The New England Journal of Medicine,* Vol. 314 (1986), pp. 605–13.

8. S. N. Blair, H. W. Kohl, R. S. Paffenbarger, D. G. Clark, K. H. Cooper, and L. W. Gibbins, "Physical Fitness and All-Cause Mortality: A Prospective Study of Healthy Men and Women," *JAMA,* Vol. 262 (1989), pp. 2395–2401.

9. S. P. Helmrich, D. R. Ragland, R. W. Lueng, and R. S. Paffenbarger, "Physical Activity and Reduced Occurrence of Non-Insulin-Dependent Diabetes Mellitus," *The New England Journal of Medicine,* Vol. 325 (1991), pp. 147–52.

10. J. W. Anderson, C. C. Hamilton, and V. Brinkman-Kaplan, "Benefits and Risks of an Intensive Very-Low-Calorie Diet Program for Severe Obesity," *American Journal of Gastroenterology,* Vol. 89 (1992), pp. 6–15.

11. C. Bouchard, J.-P. Depres, and A. Tremblay, "Exercise and Obesity," *Obesity Research,* Vol. 1 (1993), pp. 133–47.

CHAPTER 12

1. Alfred Adler, *The Practice and Theory of Individual Psychology,* trans. P. Radin (London: Kegan, Trench, Truber & Co., LTD, 1946), pp. 1–350.

2. Alfred Adler, *Social Interest: A Challenge to Mankind,* trans. John Linton and Richard Vaughan (New York: Capricorn Books, 1964), pp. 19–68.

3. Alfred Adler, *What Life Should Mean to You.* ed. Alan Porter (New York: Capricorn Books, 1958), pp. 1–300.

4. Albert Ellis and Russell Grieger, *Handbook of Rational-Emotive Therapy* (New York: Springer Publishing Co., 1977), pp. 3–35.

5. Karen Horney, *Self-Analysis* (New York: W. W. Norton, 1942), pp. 1–150.

6. Arnold A. Lazarus, "Toward an Egoless State of Being," in *Handbook of Rational-Emotive Therapy* (New York: Springer Publishing Co., 1977), pp. 113–18.

7. Arnold A. Lazarus and Allen Fay, *I Can If I Want To* (New York: William Morrow and Company, Inc., 1975), pp. 1–118.

CHAPTER 13

1. Geoffrey Cowley, "It's the Hot Sleeping Pill, Natural and Cheap. Now Scientists Say This Hormone Could Reset the Body's Aging Clock, Turning Back the Ravages of Time: Melatonin," *Newsweek* (August 7, 1995), pp. 46–49.
2. "Drug of Darkness: Can a Pineal Hormone Head Off Everything from Breast Cancer to Aging?" *Science News,* Vol. 147 (May 13, 1995), pp. 300–301.
3. R. J. Reiter, et al., "Melatonin as a Free Radical Scavenger: Implications for Aging and Age-Related Diseases," *Annals of the New York Academy of Sciences,* Vol. 719 (1994), pp. 1–12.
4. Gregory G. Mader, "Melatonin May Help Elderly Insomnics," news release (September 15, 1995) from the American Sleep Disorders Association and the Sleep Research Society about the article on this topic published in their jointly produced journal *Sleep.* The two independent organizations represent more than three thousand physicians and laboratory scientists practicing and doing sleep research in connection with pulmonary medicine, neurology, psychiatry, otolaryngology, internal medicine, pediatrics, and other medical disciplines.
5. D. Garfinkel, et al., "Improvement of Sleep Quality in Elderly People by Controlled-Release Melatonin," *Lancet,* Vol. 346 (August 1995), pp. 541–44.
6. Cowley, "It's the Hot Sleeping Pill."
7. B. Poeggeler et al., "Melatonin, Hydroxyl Radical-Mediated Oxidative Damage, and Aging: A Hypothesis," *Journal of Pineal Research,* Vol. 14 (1993), p. 157.
8. "Melatonin," *The Medical Letter,* Vol. 37 (November 24, 1995), pp. 111–12.
9. Geoffrey Cowley, "Melatonin Mania," *Newsweek* (November 6, 1995), p. 60.
10. W. Pierpaoli, W. Regelson, and C. Colman, *The Melatonin Miracle: Nature's Age-Reversing, Disease-Fighting, Sex-Enhancing Hormone* (New York: Simon & Schuster, 1995).
11. R. J. Reiter and J. Robinson, *Melatonin: Your Body's Natural Wonder Drug* (New York: Bantam, 1995).

CHAPTER 14

1. J. W. Anderson and N. J. Gustafson, *Dr. Anderson's High-Fiber Fitness Plan* (Lexington: University Press of Kentucky, 1994).

APPENDIX A

1. Interview with Dr. Stephen Barnes, a professor of pharmacology-toxicology working under American Cancer Society and National Cancer Institute grants at the University of Alabama at Birmingham.
2. Judy Shabert, *The Ultimate Nutrient Glutamine: The Essential Nonessential Amino Acid* (Garden City Park, NY: Avery, 1995), p. 51.
3. Gary E. Hatch, "Vitamin C and Asthma," *American Journal of Clinical Nutrition,* Vol. 61 (1995), pp. 625–30.

GLOSSARY

1. Editors of *Prevention* Health Books, *The Complete Book of Natural and Medicinal Cures* (Emmaus, PA: Rodale Health Books, 1994), p. 114.
2. Jean R. Hine, "Folic Acid: Contemporary Clinical Perspective," *Perspectives in Applied Nutrition,* Vol. 1, No. 2 (Autumn 1993), pp. 3–14.

GLOSSARY: ALL YOU EVER WANTED TO KNOW ABOUT FREE RADICALS AND OTHER TERMS USED IN THIS BOOK

Although we have usually defined terms as we have used them, of necessity such definitions are terse, sometimes amounting to only labels. That's why we developed this glossary, covering in greater depth the medical and nutritional terms used in this book.

Allium vegetables: Garlic, onions, and other allium family members (see Table 8.2) are rich in allicin and other sulfur-containing phytochemicals that decrease blood clotting, lower blood cholesterol levels, and protect against cancer and heart attack. Enteric-coated tablets may reduce "garlic breath."

Alpha-tocopherol: The scientific name for a component of vitamin E is tocopherol. The most biologically active form is alpha-tocopherol. A *d* before "alpha-tocopherol" means *dextra,* which is Latin for "right."

Alzheimer's disease: An incurable brain disorder characterized by a slow but inexorable deterioration of mental capacity and failure of memory. The disorder develops gradually, often starting in late middle age.

Antibodies: Any of a large number of protein molecules produced by specialized B cells after stimulation by an antigen. The B cells tailormake antibodies to fight specific antigens (see antigens in this appendix) in a process called the immune response. For example, the flu virus stimulates the production of antibodies that can attach to and destroy only that particular virus.

Antigens: These invading substances, usually bacteria or viruses, sometimes poisons or other toxic chemicals, stimulate the production of defense mechanisms called antibodies (see antibodies in this appendix).

Antioxidants: A group of elements including enzymes, vitamins, minerals, and other substances that oppose the process of oxidation (see oxidation in this appendix).

Arteriosclerosis: The medical term for hardening of the arteries caused by the process of atherosclerosis.

Artery: A muscular tube that forms part of the system of vessels that carry oxygen-rich blood from the lungs to the heart, which then pumps the bright red fluid throughout the body. Arterial blood is bright red because it has been filtered and packed with oxygen while passing through the lungs.

Atherosclerosis: This is the accumulation of gruel-like fatty compounds called foam cells on the inner lining of the coronary arteries. The foam cells coalesce, roughening the inner cell wall. This roughening can develop into a dangerous protrusion termed an atheroma. This is dangerous because the fat-filled, yellow-streaked atheroma pushes against the inner lining of the coronary artery. The increased internal pressure causes the artery to rupture, forming a thrombotic occlusion, the blocking of an artery by a clot. The rupture of the inner artery wall and resulting thrombosis causes what doctors call an infarction, what everyone else calls a heart attack.

Bile: This thick, yellowish-brown, sometimes greenish fluid contains cholesterol; other fats; bile acids; and bilirubin, a waste product resulting from red blood cell destruction. Bile acids have a detergentlike effect on fats, breaking them apart so that enzymes from the pancreas can digest the fats. This process is called emulsification, and without it, most of the fat ingested from our diets would remain undigested. If you are overweight you would probably think this is a good thing, but fat, in appropriate amounts, is needed by the body to cushion internal organs and serve as an energy reservoir. The end result of the emulsification process is that bile, containing the undigested fats and bilirubin, is then excreted, leaving the body in feces.

Bioflavonoids: See flavonoids in this appendix.

Calcium: The most abundant mineral in our bodies. Up to 98 percent of this mineral is found in our skeleton; the remaining 2 percent is in the blood and tissues. Calcium works with magnesium in regulating the contraction of muscles, most importantly the heart muscle. The substance also has a role in nerve conduction, the passage of signals along our nerve networks. Calcium is found in high amounts in milk, in many leafy vegetables such as broccoli and cauliflower, and in peas and beans such as pintos and soybeans. Nuts such as almonds, Brazil nuts, and hazelnuts, and seeds such as sunflower and sesame also contain calcium.

Capsaicin: This spicy ingredient makes cayenne and other peppers taste hot. It is also the source of most of the medicinal effects of peppers. It is considered a natural stimulant, acting as a mild diuretic and providing energy. There are about twenty species and hundreds of varieties in pepper genus *Capsicum*. In laboratory tests, capsaicin as been shown to interfere with pain signals related to the brain from skin sensory nerves. Capsaicin has been used to treat various types of pain, including the pain of arthritis.

Carcinogen: An agent, process, or substance that causes cancer.

Carotene: A substance the body uses to make vitamin A. Carotene occurs naturally in many vegetables and fruits, including apricots, cantaloupe, carrots, sweet potatoes, and spinach.

Carotenoids: These are phytochemicals and antioxidants that give color to plants. More than six hundred carotenoids are divided into two major families, carotenes and xanthophyll. Carotenes include beta-carotene and lycopene. Capsanthin in red paprika is a commonly used xanthophyll. These compounds are not toxic, as excessive intake of vitamin A can be. Many but not all carotenoids are converted to vitamin A, but only as needed by the body. Virtually all carotenoids have antioxidant properties: High blood levels of these phytochemicals are usually associated with lowered risks of disease. One recent study, for instance, showed that men with high blood levels of carotenoids had a one-third lower risk of heart disease, even when their blood cholesterol levels were high, than a similar group of other men.

Catechins: These are major antioxidants in green tea. Black and oolong tea contain similar compounds that have been slightly modified during the processing of the tea leaves.

Cruciferous vegetables: This family of vegetables includes broccoli, Brussels sprouts, cabbage, cauliflower, radishes, turnips, and watercress. They are rich in indoles (substances made by the human body), isothiocyanates (see isothiocyanates in this appendix), and also are packed full of phytochemicals that protect against cancer. (See Chapter 4 and Table 4.1.)

Diabetes: In this disease, cells of the body have an impaired ability to recognize and burn sugar (glucose) needed for energy. Uncontrolled diabetes leads to fatigue and ultimately to death.

DNA: The abbreviation for deoxyribonucleic acid. It is the genetic material within our chromosomes that regulates the life activities of each cell.

Electron: An elementary particle or unit of negative electricity. All atoms have electrons surrounding a nucleus. When an atom loses an electron, it becomes a free radical (see free radicals in this appendix).

Ellagic acid: One of the important antioxidants in red wine that protect against heart attack.

Enzymes: A complex protein compound produced by living cells that causes or speeds up chemical reactions in other substances. For instance, the enzyme pepsin helps break down food so it can be digested. More than a thousand different enzymes have been identified in the human body.

FABB: Folic Acid and Vitamins B_6 and B_{12}. These water-soluble vitamins lower the chemical homocysteine in the blood, thereby protecting the cardiovascular system.

Faustian bargain: A German legend tells about an astrologer named Faust who made a pact with the devil, surrendering his soul in return for youth, knowledge, and magical power. A Faustian bargain is acceptance of something bad later in life for immediate benefits.

Flavonoids (also called bioflavonoids): This large group of nutrients, produced by many plants, are essential for the proper absorption of vitamin C. They also help vitamin C keep collagen, the "glue" that holds cells together, healthy. Bioflavonoids act as antioxidants by protecting vitamin C from free-radical-caused oxidation. Flavonoids occur naturally in vegetables, fruits, tea, and wine. More than four thousand chemically unique phytochemicals in this category have been identified. As outlined in Chapter 3, the intake of flavonoids from tea, onions, apples, and other foods is associated with a significant reduction in heart attack rates in the Netherlands. Flavonoids appear to lower the incidence of coronary disease, perhaps by lowering cholesterol. Other good sources of flavonoids include apricots, beans, black currants, cherries, cola nuts, cranberries, grapefruit, grapes, lemons, plums, and rose hips.

Folic acid: The term folic, from the Latin *folium,* which means "leaf," is appropriate because this nutrient is found in green leaves (as well as in animal tissues). This B-complex component is involved in many bodily processes, including protein metabolism and cell division and replication (see Chapters 3 and 8). Doctors now know that women of childbearing age should take a 0.4-mg dose of folic acid to prevent birth defects. In 1992 the Centers for Disease Control and the U.S. Public Health Service recommended that women of childbearing age ingest 0.4 mg of folic acid daily to protect against birth defects.[2]

Free radicals: Organic compounds that have lost one or some other odd number of electrons. Having an unpaired electron makes a free radical unstable, causing it to seek out a mate.

Free radical scavengers: A term used interchangeably with antioxidants.

Glucose: A simple sugar that is carried in the blood to the cells. The hormone insulin "unlocks" the cell membrane, allowing glucose to penetrate into the cell. Once within, mitochondria (see mitochondria in this appendix) burn glucose to provide the body's chief source of energy.

Homocysteine: This naturally occurring amino acid plays an important role in regulating the body's metabolism. Vitamins' B6, B12, and folic acid help regulate the levels of homocysteine in the blood. People who fail to get enough of these vitamins may have high blood levels of homocysteine. High levels damage blood vessels and are linked to cardiovascular disease and stroke and may also be involved in cancer and other age-related health problems. The best dietary sources of these three vitamins are green, leafy vegetables, whole grains, and nuts.

Hormones: Hormones (from a Greek word that means "urge on") regulate many varied functions within cells and tissues. One hormone stimulates the maturation of the sex organs and another the growth of bones. Still another controls the metabolic rate of the cells. Hormones work by grasping receptors, recognition sites of various tissues on which hormones act. Insulin is one such hormone.

Humulin: Brand name of an insulin manufactured using recombinant DNA technology by Eli Lilly & Company. This insulin is structurally identical to the insulin produced by the human body.

Immune system: The Latin term *immuno* means *protection,* and that's what the immune system tries to do for our bodies. The immune system is a network of protective mechanisms that produce defenders, such as antibodies, that battle against invading infectious diseases, viruses, or parasites. However, when the immune system is overextended and overwhelmed, it becomes confused, creating disturbances called autoimmune disorders, which cause inflammation and body cell injuries. Antioxidants act like reinforcements of soldiers and paramedics, strengthening the immune system and keeping it from being overwhelmed by the sickness-causing invaders.

Indoles: Broccoli and other cruciferous vegetables contain phytochemicals that your body changes into indoles. Indoles protect the body against cancer. (See Chapter 4 and Table 4.1.)

Insulin: A hormone made up of fifty-one amino acids secreted by the islet cells of the pancreas. Insulin lowers the amount of glucose in the blood by transferring this simple sugar into cells, where the glucose is burned for energy. Insulin also helps the liver convert and store glucose both in the liver and in muscles as a form of a starch known as glycogen. In addition, insulin helps the body repair tissue and store fat.

Isoflavones: Soy products are major sources of isoflavones such as genistein (see Appendix A) and daidzein, which have many protective properties as outlined in Chapter 7.

Isothiocyanates: Broccoli and other cruciferous vegetables (See Table 8.2) are rich in these phytochemicals which protect the body against a number of different forms of cancer (see Chapter 4 and Table 4.1).

Limonene: A phytochemical and antioxidant that comes from citrus fruit. It reduces the risk of several types of cancer.

Lipids: Fatty substances found in foods and in the body. In the body, lipids are sources of stored energy, but they can also build up within blood vessels, causing dangerous internal pressures and blockages. Examples of lipids include cholesterol and triglycerides.

Lipoprotein: Fatty substances called lipids bound together with protein are called lipoproteins. High levels of low-density lipoproteins (LDL) are associated with atherosclerosis (see atherosclerosis in this appendix) and increased risk of heart attack. High levels of high-density lipoproteins (HDL) are found in persons who are at less risk for atherosclerosis.

Macrophages: Cells located in the spleen and bone marrow that clean up and digest worn-out red blood cells. They are categorized as histiocytes or phagocytic cells because they protect the body by engulfing foreign materials.

Melatonin: A hormone secreted by the pineal gland that contributes to skin pigmentation. See Chapter 13, "Melatonin Update," and Appendix A, "Antioxidant and Phytochemical Advisory," for more information.

Membrane: A very thin but relatively strong and pliable sheet of tissue that covers and connects cells and tissues.

Metabolism: The sum total of the chemical processes in living organisms that allow growth, production of energy, and the maintenance of vital functions of living. Metabolism is the "sum total" of these chemical processes because it includes anabolism, (the building up of the body) and catabolism (the process in which used-up cells and tissues are broken down, used for energy, and then excreted).

Mitochondria: Tiny, energy-producing factories within each cell. The mitochondria create energy by burning food in the presence of oxygen.

Molecule: An element consisting of two or more atoms. Molecular substances can exist as gases, liquids, or solids.

Nerve cells: Microscopic cells collected into bundles called *nerves* carry electrical and chemical messages all over the body. External stimuli (such as a touch or an aroma) and internal stimuli (hormones, prostaglandins, and other chemicals) activate nerve cell membranes, causing them to release stored electrical energy. When released, that energy, a *nerve impulse,* travels the length of the cell and chemically jumps the space between it and other nerve cells. External receptors on these other cells receive and forward these impulses to the complex network of cells in the brain and spinal cord known as the central nervous system (CNS). The CNS is where nerve impulses are recognized, interpreted, and rapidly relayed (quicker than a blink of the eye) to their destination, other nerve cells in almost any part of the body. The message may trigger a conscious thought or a subconscious physical response such as a yawn.

Neurologist: A medical doctor who specializes in diseases of the brain and central nervous system.

Organsulfur compounds: Sulfur-containing phytochemicals found in allium vegetables. These compounds have a number of positive health effects, including providing protection against cancer and heart disease.

Osteoarthritis: Also called degenerative joint disease, osteoarthritis is the most prevalent form of arthritis in the United States.

Oxidation: A circular process of change, specifically burning or rusting. In this process, atoms, ions, or molecules change by losing electrons. This process provides needed energy for life, but also produces free radicals, which, in turn, also burn into cells and tissues, continuing the oxidation process.

Oxygen: This odorless, colorless, and tasteless gas makes up by volume one-fifth of the atmosphere. Humans, animals, plants, and most other organisms cannot live without oxygen. The prestigious journal *Scientific American* states: "Oxygen is our chief source of energy, being responsible for the respiration of living organisms and the combustion of fuels."

Pancreas: A large, somewhat hammer-shaped gland located in front of the upper lumbar vertebrae and behind the stomach. Throughout the pancreas are tiny islands known as the *islets of Langerhans* (for the German doctor who discovered them) which include *beta cells*. These cells, which total less than 1 percent of the volume of the entire pancreas, manufacture life-giving insulin, which passes directly into the bloodstream. The remainder of the pancreas is devoted to secreting digestive juices into the duodenum, the first part of the small intestine.

Parkinson's disease: A slowly progressive, degenerative brain disease occurring in later life. Degeneration of the nerves in the brain and central nervous system leads to resting tremors, weakness and rigidity of muscles, a shuffling gait, and postural instability. It is thought that damage to small areas of the midbrain may be the result of viral infections or cerebral arteriosclerosis. Some drugs are temporarily useful in controlling symptoms, but the disease itself is incurable. There is evidence that antioxidants early in life may protect against the development of Parkinson's disease later in life.

Pharmacologist: An expert trained to study the preparation, properties, uses, and effects of drugs.

Phenolic compounds: This large category of phytochemicals include caffeic acid and ferulic acid from blueberries, grapes, oats, prunes, and soybeans; catechins from tea; curcumin from mustard and turmeric; ellagic acid from grapes, raspberries, and strawberries; quercetin from cereal grains, coffee, onions, and tea; sesamol from sesame seeds; and vanillin from cloves and vanilla beans. These phytochemicals protect against cancer and heart disease.

Phytic acid: This phosphorus-containing acid is present in the outer layer of most cereal grains, nuts, and beans. When ingested it may interfere with the intestinal absorption of various minerals, especially calcium and magnesium.

Phytochemicals: Literally, chemicals produced by plants.

Polypeptide: A compound of many amino acids linked in a particular manner.

Prostaglandins: A class of physiologically active, hormonelike substances first found in semen (which is made in the prostate, hence the name). These substances, now known to be found in many body cells, work to lower blood pressure, regulate body temperature, aid stomach acid secretion, and stimulate contractions of the uterus. Prostaglandins also work to relieve inflammation, but they encourage the production of free radicals and thus can be considered a "two-edged sword."

Protease: Any of numerous enzymes that hydrolyze (help us digest) protein. Also called proteinase.

Protease inhibitors: Pinto and navy beans contain chemicals that inhibit the protese enzymes, which help us digest protein.

Red blood cells: The formal name for these cells is erythrocytes. Erythrocytes are made in the bone marrow and are important because they transport oxygen from the lungs through the bloodstream to cells all over the body. The oxygen is then used by the cells as they convert food to energy. Erythrocytes also carry away carbon dioxide, a waste product of the energy production in the cells. An important protein in erythrocytes that helps carry the oxygen as it travels through the bloodstream is hemoglobin. (Hemo for heme, an iron-containing red compound, and globin, a colorless protein).

Sclerosis: The process of hardening of a tissue, vessel, or other part of the body.

Serum cholesterol: Fatty lipoproteins found in the serum or blood. Lipoproteins are fat (lipids) and protein molecules bound together. There are "good guy" and "bad guy" lipoproteins. (See lipoprotein in this appendix.)

Sulfurophane: This sulfur-containing phytochemical is also found in many vegetables and has protective effects against cancer.

T cells: Created by the thymus gland, T cells protect the body in at least five ways. They: (1) attach to antigens and destroy them; (2) stimulate cells called macrophages to recognize and ingest antigens; (3) secrete proteins that help other cells respond to antigens; (4) act as helper cells to promote the creation of antibodies; and (5) act as suppressor cells to inhibit the creation of unwarranted antibodies. (Too many antibodies, or antibodies created at the wrong time, can cause the immune system to attack its own host.)

Thymus: A small, glandlike organ found near the base of the neck. Not to be confused with the thyroid gland, also in the neck. While the thyroid gland affects growth and metabolism, the thymus is essential for the early development and later functioning of the human immune system. The thymus produces T cells, which battle bacteria, viruses, fungi, and parasites that attempt to invade the body. This organ starts shrinking shortly after puberty and produces fewer and fewer T cells as we age.

Triglycerides: Sweet, fatty substances, the results of digestion. As the prefix "tri" indicates, a triglyceride molecule has three fatty acid molecules to every one molecule of glycerol.

White blood cells: The number of certain varieties of these cells, all of which are technically called leukocytes, provides an indication of how strong our immune systems are. There are five kinds of leukocytes, divided into two major groups, granulocytes and agranulocytes. Granulocytes are the most numerous leukocytes (60 percent). This group includes basophils, eosinophils, and neutrophiles. Neutrophiles, which compose 57 percent of all leukocytes, fight disease by engulfing and swallowing up germs. The two other types of granulocytes—basophils and eosinophils—appear in great numbers when we are sick. The exact function of basophils is unknown, but their numbers increase in leukemia. Eosinophils increase in number when the body suffers an allergic condition or a parasitic infection. Agranulocytes, the second major group of leukocytes, is made up of two types, lymphocytes and monocytes. Lymphocytes (about 33 percent of all leukocytes) make *antibodies*, which destroy *antigens* (see antibodies and antigens in this appendix). Monocytes, also called macrophages, dispose of dead and dying cells by engulfing and swallowing them.

INDEX

A

Adler, Alfred, 195

Adult-onset diabetes, *see* Type II diabetes

Aerobic, upper-body exercise, 126, 134–35, 142, 173, 179–80, 181, 215–16

Age-related macular degeneration (ARMD), 11, 18, 101, 103, 104

Aging, 21–33, 87–88
  antioxidant, antiaging program and, 22–33, 88
  antioxidants and, 5, 6, 9, 11, 12, 18, 28–29
  diet and, 118, 126
  exercise and, 126
  free radicals and, 7, 8, 17, 92
  free radical, wear-and-tear theory of, 92
  genetic theory of, 25–26
  health-promoting habits and, 127
  immunologic theory of, 23–24
  melatonin and, 25, 138, 207
  metabolic theory of, 24–25
  phytochemicals and, 5, 6, 11, 12, 18
  soy protein and, 118
  supplements and, 126
  theories of, 23–28
  thymus and, 23–24
  vitamin E and, 26
  wear-and-tear, free radical theory of, 26–28
  see also Arthritis; Brain; Diabetes; Eye diseases; Skin

Alcohol, recommendations on, 141, 190, 215

Allison's new french toast, 144

Allium vegetables, 60, 129

Allyl sulfides, cancer and, 59, 60

Alpha-tocopherol, *see* Vitamin E

Alzheimer, Alois, 77

Alzheimer's disease, 75, 77–78
  antioxidants and, 11, 18, 28
  brain stimulation and, 81
  free radicals and, 27, 28
  melatonin and, 138, 207
  phytochemicals and, 11, 18

American Cancer Society (ACS), 67–68

Ames, Bruce, 12

Amyloid protein, Alzheimer's disease and, 77–78

Anemia, iron supplements and, 136

Angier, Natalie, 7

Angina, vitamin E and, 44

Angiogenesis, soy protein and, 110

Ankylosing spondylitis, 92
  see also Arthritis

Antidepressants, 141

Antioxidant and Phytochemical advisory, 219–25

Antioxidant, antiaging food plan, *see* Diet

Antioxidant, antiaging program
  benefits of, 11–12, 18
  levels, 18–19, *see also* Disease reversal; General prevention; Tailored protection
  stage 1 of, 213–15
  stage 2 of, 215–16
  stage 3 of, 216–17
  see also Diet; Exercise; Supplements

Antioxidants, 5, 6, 8
  age-related macular degeneration
    and, 103, 104
  aging and, 5, 6, 9, 11, 12, 18, 28–29
  Alzheimer's disease and, 11, 18, 28
  animal studies of, 41
  Antioxidant and Phytochemical
    advisory, 219–25
  arteriosclerosis and, 11, 18
  arthritis and, 11, 18, 92–93
  brain and, 74, 75–76, 78, 79–80
  cancer and, 11, 18, 28–29, 54–55,
    57–59, 61–69
  cataracts and, 11, 18, 103–4
  cells producing, 9
  cholesterol and, 15, 16
  classes and compounds of, 219–25
  definition, 9, 219
  diabetes and, 11, 18, 98–101
  eye diseases and, 11, 18, 103–4
  flavonoids, 45–46, 53
  food sources of, 53, 128, 129, 185,
    187, see also Vegetables and fruits
  free radicals and, 4, 5, 10
  function of, 9–10
  heart attack and, 11, 18
  heart disease and, 28–29, 35, 40–46
  human studies of, 41
  hunter-gatherers and, 4–5
  immune system and, 24, 29–31
  low-density lipoproteins and, 40–46
  osteoporosis and, 11, 18
  Parkinson's disease and, 28
  skin and, 90–91
  stroke and, 11, 18
  supplements, 127, 135–37, 142, 213
  weight loss and, 13–14
  see also Beta-carotene; Diet;
    Isoflavones; Vitamin C; Vitamin E
Apples
  apple pancakes, 145
  apple soy muffins, 147
  shopping for, 186
Apricot pumpkin bread, 148
Aretaeus of Cappadocia, 77
Arteries, hardening of the, see
  Arteriosclerosis

Arteriosclerosis, 38, 39
  antioxidant, antiaging program and,
    35–36, 40–46
  antioxidants and, 11, 18
  cholesterol and, 47
  definition, 36
  fat and, 47
  free radicals and, 8
  heart attack and, 36–40
  low-density lipoproteins and, 40–47
  phytochemicals and, 11, 18
  stroke and, 36–40
  tailored protection and, 50
Arthritis, 91–93
  antioxidants and, 11, 18, 92–93
  free radicals and, 27, 92, 93
  phytochemicals and, 11, 18
Arts, brain stimulated with, 84
Aspirin
  enteric-coated, 51, 138
  fibrinogen and, 49
  recommended daily intake of, 126,
    138, 142, 213
Atheroma, 38–39, 40
Atherosclerosis, free radicals and, 26
  see also Arteriosclerosis
Avocados, shopping for, 186
Axons, 81

B

Bacteria, free radicals and, 10
Baked beans, Belinda's, 156
Bananas
  banana nut soy muffins, 149
  shopping for, 186
Bark, Joseph P., 89
Beans, 188–89
  Belinda's baked, 156
  benefits of, 188
  black bean dip, 169
  cancer and, 59, 60
  down home chili, 164
  shopping for, 188–89
Belinda's baked beans, 156
Berries, shopping for, 186
Beta-carotene, 17, 63

Beta-carotene (*cont.*)
  amount of in diet, 52
  benefits of, 142
  cancer and, 54, 55, 58, 59, 60, 62,
    64–68
  cataracts and, 104
  cholesterol and, 16
  definition, 6
  food sources of, 45, 53, 57, 185
  heart attack and, 42, 44–45
  heart disease and, 34
  recommended daily intake of, 127,
    136, 142, 219–20
  supplements, 45, 52, 55
  vegetables and fruits containing,
    129, 226–28
Beverages
  shopping for, 190
  strawberry-banana frosty, 170
  tangy vegetable juice, 171
  tutti-fruitti, 170
  see also Tea
Biological clock, pineal gland as, 138,
    204
Black beans, 189
  black bean dip, 169
Black tea, 141, 224–25
  see also Green tea
Blair, S. N., 176
Blindness, free radicals and, 27
Block, Gladys, 62
Blood pressure
  exercise and, 177
  heart disease and, 48, 49
Blueberry soy muffins, 150
Blumberg, Jeffrey, 26, 30, 66
Bogden, John, 30–31
Brain, 27, 73–86
  antioxidants and, 74, 75–76, 78,
    79–80
  diet and, 85
  free radicals and, 75, 76, 77, 79
  memory loss and, 73–74, *see also*
    Alzheimer's disease
  mental calisthenics and, 80–83, 86
  slowing loss of cells and, 74–76
  stimulation of, 80–84

supplements and, 85
  see also Parkinson's disease
Breads
  apricot pumpkin, 148
  shopping for, 190
Breakfast
  menu plans for, 132
  recipes for, 144–51, 170
  in restaurants, 191
  worksheet for increasing antioxidant
    foods in, 130
Breast cancer, 55, 60, 208
  soy protein and, 12, 63, 109, 110,
    111, 115–17, 121, 221
  tamoxifen and, 110–11, 117
  see also Cancer
Broccoli
  gingered broccoli with pasta, 160–
    61
  health benefits of, 129

C

Caffeine, 141, 190
Calcium
  free radicals and, 8
  supplements and osteoporosis
    prevention and, 136
Calories, in diet, 133, 134
Cancer
  antioxidant, antiaging program and,
    34–53
  antioxidants and, 11, 18, 28–29,
    54–55, 57–59, 61–69
  beta-carotene and, 55, 58, 59, 60,
    62, 220
  diet and, 70, 71, 126
  exercise and, 71, 126, 175, 176
  free radicals and, 7, 8, 17, 26
  garlic and, 221
  general prevention and, 70
  health-promoting habits and, 127
  initiation phase of, 58
  lung, 55, 63, 68
  melatonin and, 207–8
  phytochemicals and, 11, 18, 56–61
  progression phase of, 59

Cancer (*cont.*)
  promotion phase of, 58
  reversal of, 71
  selenium and, 54, 55, 62, 63, 68
  soy protein and, 12, 59, 107–8, 109,
    110, 111, 115–17, 121, 221
  stomach, 58, 63
  supplements and, 54–55, 63–69, 70,
    71, 126
  tailored protection and, 71
  in the United States, 55–56
  vegetables and fruits and, 60, 61–63,
    68
  vitamin C and, 58, 59–60, 62, 63
  vitamin E and, 54, 55, 58, 62, 63, 68
  See also Breast cancer; Colon cancer;
    Prostate cancer
"Can do" attitude, motivation
    strengthened by, 194, 198
Cardiovascular disease, vitamin B
    supplements and, 46
  see also Heart attack; Heart disease;
    Stroke
Carney, John M., 28
Carotene and Retinol Efficacy Trial
    (CARET), 65–66, 67
Carrots
  curried carrot soup, 154
  glazed snow peas and carrots, 157
Cataracts, 11, 18, 102, 103–4
Catechins, cancer and, 60, 61
Cell death, calcium overload and, 8
Cereals, shopping for, 190
Chandra, Ranjit K., 29–30
Chemoprevention, cancer and, 56
  phytochemicals and, 56–61
Chickpeas, 189
Chili, down home, 164
China, antioxidant supplements and
    cancer protection in, 54–55, 63,
    68, 72
Chocolate pudding, soy-good, 171
Cholesterol
  antioxidant, antiaging program and,
    15–17, 21, 34, 35
  arteriosclerosis and, 47
  desirable levels of, 47–48
  diet and, 15–16
  garlic and, 221
  heart disease and, 36–40, 51
  positive purposes of, 37
  soy protein and, 12, 110, 111,
    112–15, 117–18
  stroke and, 36–40
  test of, 51, 52
  vitamin E and, 16, 109
  See also High-density lipoproteins;
    Low-density lipoproteins;
    Very-low-density lipoproteins
Christian, William, Jr., 102
Chromium, 220–21
Chylomicrons, 47
Cigarettes, *see* Nonsmoking; Smoking
Citrus spinach salad, 152
Citrus surprise, 146
Clarkson, Tom, 114
Coenzyme Q, 221
Coffee, 141, 190
Collins, James, 103
Colon cancer, 55, 63, 220
  aspirin and, 138
  soy protein and, 111
  see also Cancer
Cooper, Kenneth H., 31, 173
Crackers, shopping for, 190
Creamy spinach soup, 155
Crofford, Oscar, 98
Cross-training, *see* Upper-body
    exercise; Walking
Crow's-feet, 89
Cruciferous vegetables, 60, 129
Curried carrot soup, 154

D

Daidzein, 12, 60, 61, 110, 221, 222
  see also Isoflavones
Degenerative joint disease, *see* Arthritis
De León, Ponce, 142
Dementias of the Alzheimer type
    (DAT), 78
Dendrites, 81
De Soto, Hernando, 142
Desserts, recipes for, 146, 171–72

Diabetes, 94–101
  antioxidant, antiaging program and,
    21–22, 32–33, 34, 41, 94–101
  antioxidants and, 11, 18, 98–100
  causes of, 96
  danger of, 95, 96
  diet and, 94–95, 97, 99–101
  exercise and, 94–95, 96–97, 177
  eye disease and, 99, 106
  fat and, 100
  free radicals and, 27, 96, 98, 99
  heart disease and, 48, 49, 96
  high-fiber diet and, 100–101
  kidney damage and, 99
  phytochemicals and, 11, 18
  Type I, 97
  Type II, 97–98, 99–100, 177
Diabetes Control and Complications
    Trial (DCCT), 97, 98
Diet, 25, 53, 141–42
  aging and, 118, 126
  brain function and, 85
  calories in, 133, 134
  cancer and, 70, 71, 126
  cholesterol and, 15–16
  diabetes and, 94–95, 97, 99–100
  disease reversal and, 126
  general prevention and, 126
  heart disease and, 51, 52, 126
  high-fiber, 47, 100–101, 141
  low-density lipoproteins and, 47
  menu plans, 132–34
  stages of implementing, 214–15,
    216, 217
  tailored protection and, 126
  weight loss and, 12–14, 17
  worksheet for increasing antioxidant
    foods in, 130–31
  see also Antioxidants; Recipes; Soy
    protein; Vegetables and fruits
Diet sodas, 190
Digitalis, 110
Dinner
  menu plans for, 133, 134
  recipes for, 152–69
  worksheet for increasing antioxidant
    foods in, 131
Dip, black bean, 169

Diplock, Anthony T., 31
Disease reversal, 18–19
  cancer and, 71
  diet and, 126
  exercise and, 126, 179, 181
  health-promoting habits and, 127
  heart disease and, 52
  program for, 126–28
  serum lipids level and, 47, 48
  soy protein and, 122
  supplements and, 126, 127, 137
DNA, free radicals and, 8, 9, 10, 17
Down home chili, 164

E

Ears, calisthenics and, 82
Easy vegetable primavera, 163
Ehrenberg, Miriam, 81–82
Ehrenberg, Otto, 82
Ellagic acid, cancer and, 60, 61
Ellis, Albert, 195
Emerit, Ingrid, 90–91
Enstrom, J. E., 45
Environmental pollutants, 4
Estradiole, soy protein compared to,
    110–11, 117–18
Estrogen, 60
Estrogen replacement, soy protein
    instead of, 116, 118
Exercise, 52, 173–84, 217
  aging and, 126
  benefits of, 174
  blood pressure and, 177
  brain and, 80–83, 86
  cancer and, 70, 71, 126, 176
  cholesterol and, 15–16
  diabetes and, 94–95, 96–97, 177
  disease reversal and, 126, 179,
    181
  free radicals and, 6, 174, 185
  general prevention and, 126, 179,
    181
  heart disease and, 35, 51, 52, 126,
    175–76
  high-density lipoproteins and, 47
  high-intensity, 6

Exercise (*cont.*)
  recommended amount of, 174,
    178–80, 181
  tailored protection and, 126, 179,
    181
  upper-body, 126, 134–35, 142, 173,
    179–80, 181, 215–16
  walking, 126, 134, 135, 142, 173,
    178–80, 181–82, 183, 195–96,
    214
  weight loss/control and, 13, 14, 178,
    179–80
Eye diseases, 101–4
  age-related macular degeneration,
    11, 18, 101, 103, 104
  antioxidants and, 11, 18, 103–4
  blindness, 27
  cataracts, 11, 18, 102, 103–4
  diabetes and, 99, 106
  eye protection and, 106
  free radicals and, 27, 101
  medications and, 106
  phytochemicals and, 11, 18
  supplements and, 104–5
Eyes, exercise and, 82

F

FABB supplement
  homocysteine level and, 46, 52, 137
  recommended daily intake of, 126,
    137, 213
Fahn, Stanley, 80
Fat
  arteriosclerosis and, 47
  desirable levels of, 47–48
  diabetes and, 100
  food sources of, 47
  heart attack/stroke and, 36–40
  positive purposes of, 37
  recommended daily intake of, 126
Fiber, 100
  food sources of, 185
  high-fiber diet, 47, 100–101, 141
  recommended daily intake of, 126
Fibrinogen
  aspirin and, 49

  heart disease and, 48, 49
Finnish male smokers, research on
    supplements for, 64–65, 66, 68
Fish oil, recommended daily intake of,
    127, 137, 143, 213
Fish, recommended daily intake of,
    126
Flavonoids, 45–46, 53
Foam cells, heart attack and, 37–40
Folic acid, 46, 137
  thymus and, 24
  see also FABB supplement
Food plan, *see* Diet
Free radicals, 7–8
  aging and, 8, 17
  Alzheimer's disease and, 27, 28,
    77
  antioxidants and, 4, 5, 10
  arteriosclerosis and, 8, 26
  arthritis and, 27, 92, 93
  bacteria and viruses and, 10
  body damage from, 4, 8
  brain and, 75, 76, 77, 79
  cancer and, 7, 8, 17, 26
  cataracts and, 102
  definition, 4
  diabetes and, 27, 96, 98, 99
  DNA and, 8, 9, 10, 17
  exercise and, 6, 174, 185
  eye diseases and, 27, 101–2
  formation of, 7–8
  heart attack/stroke and, 36, 38, 39
  lipid peroxidation and, 8
  Parkinson's disease and, 27–28, 79
  protection from, *see* Antioxidants;
    Phytochemicals
  protection provided by, 24
  skin aging and, 89, 90
Free radical, wear-and-tear theory of
    aging, 26–28, 92
French toast, Allison's new, 144
Fruits, *see* Vegetables and fruits

G

Games, brain stimulated with, 84
Garbanzo beans, 189

Garfinkel, D., 203
Garlic
  cancer and, 59, 60
  health benefits of, 129, 221
  recommended daily intake of, 126, 221
Gazpacho, 153–54
General prevention, 18
  cancer and, 70
  diet and, 126
  exercise and, 126, 179, 181
  health-promoting habits and, 127
  heart disease and, 51
  lipid level and, 47, 48
  soy protein and, 121
  supplements and, 126, 127, 136–37
Genetic clocks, 25
Genetic theory of aging, 25–26
Genistein, 12, 59, 60, 61, 110–11, 116, 221–22
  see also Isoflavones
Gey, K. F., 42, 43
Gilchrest, Barbara, 90
Gingered broccoli with pasta, 160–61
Ginkgo biloba, 222
Ginseng, 222
Glazed snow peas and carrots, 157
Glutamine, 222–23
Glutathione (GSH), 223
Grapes, *see* Purple grapes
Green tea, 46, 60, 61, 72, 141, 190, 224–25

H

Hand work, brain and, 84
Hardening of the arteries, *see* Arteriosclerosis
Hayflick, Leonard, 25, 26
HDLs, *see* High-density lipoproteins
Health-promoting habits, 217
  disease reversal and, 127
  general prevention and, 127
  moderation, 127, 140–41, 215
  nonsmoking, 127, 139–40, 215
  rest and relaxation, 127, 140, 215
  seat belts, 127, 140, 215

tailored protection and, 127
Heart attack, 34
  antioxidant, antiaging program and, 34, 35, 43, 44–46
  antioxidants and, 11, 18
  aspirin and, 138
  beta-carotene and, 42, 44–45
  causes of, 36–40
  definition, 36
  free radicals and, 7, 36, 38, 39
  phytochemicals and, 11, 18
  see also Heart disease
Heart disease
  antioxidant, antiaging program and, 34–53
  antioxidants and, 28–29, 35, 40–46
  beta-carotene and, 34
  blood pressure and, 38, 39
  cholesterol and, 36–40, 51
  diabetes and, 48, 49, 96
  diet and, 51, 52, 126
  exercise and, 35, 51, 52, 126, 175–76
  fibrinogen and, 48, 49
  fish oil and, 137
  foods protecting against, 51, 52, 126, *see also* Diet; Soy protein; Vegetables and fruits
  garlic reducing, 221
  general prevention and, 51
  health-promoting habits and, 127
  homocysteine and, 46, 48, 49
  nonlipid risk factors and, 48–49
  obesity and, 48, 49
  reversal of, 52
  soy protein and, 12, 107–8, 112, 114, 121, 221
  stress and, 48, 49
  supplements and, 34, 51, 52, 126
  tailored protection and, 51–52
  vitamin C and, 34, 40, 42, 45
  vitamin E and, 29, 34, 40, 42, 43, 44, 48
  see also Heart attack
High blood pressure, *see* Blood pressure

High-density lipoproteins (HDLs),
    37
    desirable levels of, 47–48
    exercise and, 47
    nonsmoking and, 47
    protective function of, 46–47
High-fiber diet, 47, 100–101, 141
Holmes, Oliver Wendell, 87
Homocysteine
    FABB supplement and, 46, 52, 137
    heart disease and, 46, 48, 49
Horney, Karen, 195

I

Immune system
    antioxidants and, 24, 29–31
    cancer and, 59
    supplements and, 29–30
Immunologic theory of aging, 23–24
Immunotherapy, cancer and, 59
Inactivity, heart disease and, 48, 49
Indoles, cancer and, 60
Initiation phase, of cancer, 58
Insomnia, melatonin and, 201, 202–7,
    210
Insulin, 96, 97
    see also Diabetes
Iron supplements, 136
Irradiation, avoidance of, 4
Isoflavones, 12, 17–18, 53, 63, 109–11,
    112, 116, 117, 118
    cancer and, 60, 61, 63
    daidzein, 12, 60, 61, 110, 221,
        222
    genistein, 12, 59, 60, 61, 110–11,
        116, 221–22
    supplements, 120
    see also Soy protein
Isothiocyanates, cancer and, 60

J

Jacques, Paul F., 103
Jet lag, melatonin and, 204, 205–6,
    210
Juice, see Vegetable juice

K

Kaminski, Michael S., 104
Kandaswami, C., 139
Kardinaal, A. F. M., 42, 44
Kidney damage, diabetes and, 99
Kiwi fruit, shopping for, 186–87

L

Lasagna, vegetarian, 162
Lazarus, Arnold, 195
LDLs, see Low-density lipoproteins
Lentils, 189
Lima beans, 188–89
Limonene, cancer and, 59–60
Lipids, 37
    in brain, 76
    free radicals and, 8
    general prevention and, 47, 48
    peroxidation, 8
    see also Triglycerides
Lipoproteins, 37
    see also High-density lipoproteins;
        Low-density lipoproteins;
        Very-low-density lipoproteins
Liver spots, 89
Low-density lipoproteins (LDLs), 37,
    38, 39, 40
    arteriosclerosis and, 40–47
    desirable levels of, 47–48
    diabetes and, 96
    low-fat, high-fiber diet and, 47
Lunch
    menu plans for, 132
    recipes for, 152–69
    worksheet for increasing antioxidant
        foods in, 130, 131
Lung cancer, 55, 63, 68
    see also Cancer
Lycopene, 223

M

Macrophages, 37, 38
Macular degeneration, see Age-related
    macular degeneration

Marinara sauce, 161
Mayne, S. T., 62, 63
Melatonin, 200–211
    aging and, 25, 138, 207
    Alzheimer's disease and, 207
    cancer and, 207–8
    experiences of authors on, 205–7
    jet lag and, 204, 205–6, 210
    recommended daily intake of, 126,
        138, 143, 210, 213, 223
    for shift workers, 204–5
    as sleeping aid, 201, 202–7, 210
    thymus and, 24
    warnings on, 208–9
Melons, shopping for, 186
Memory loss, 73–74
    see also Alzheimer's disease; Brain
Mendez, Cristobol, 173
Menéndez de Avilés, Pedro, 142
Menstrual periods, iron supplements
        and, 136
Mental calisthenics, for brain, 80–83,
    86
Menu plans, 132–34
    see also Diet
Metabolic Research Group, 100
Metabolic theory of aging, 24–25
Meydani, Simin Nikbin, 30
Mineral supplements, recommended
        daily intake of, 127, 136, 142,
        213, 219
Mitochondria, 8
Moderation, recommendations for,
        127, 140–41, 215
Motivation, 193–99
    "can do" attitude for, 194, 198
    goals for, 194
    self-talk for, 195–96, 199
    visualization strengthening,
        196–98
Muffins
    apple soy, 147
    banana nut soy, 149
    blueberry soy, 150
    super-easy your choice, 151
Mutations, free radicals causing, 8, 9,
    10

N

National Academy of Sciences, cancer
        and, 56
National Cancer Institute (NCI), 56
    Carotene and Retinol Efficacy Trial
        of, 65–66, 67
Nervous system, *see* Brain
Neurons, 81
Nicklaus, Jack, 197
Non-insulin-dependent diabetes
        (NIDDM), *see* Type II diabetes
Nonsmoking, 4
    high-density lipoproteins and, 46
    recommendations for, 127, 139–40,
        215
    see also Smoking
Nose, calisthenics and, 82–83
Nuts, recommended daily intake of,
    126

O

Obesity, heart disease and, 48, 49
    see also Weight loss/control
Omega-3 fatty acids, 137
Onions
    cancer and, 59, 60
    health benefits of, 129
Optimum Brain Power (Ehrenberg and
        Ehrenberg), 81–82
Oranges, shopping for, 186
Osteoarthritis, *see* Arthritis
Osteoporosis
    antioxidants and, 11, 18
    calcium supplement and, 136
    phytochemicals and, 11, 18
    soy protein and, 12, 107–8, 111, 117
Oxidation, free radical chain, 7
    see also Free radicals
Oxygen, 7, 8

P

Packer, Lester, 25–26, 28
Pancakes, apple, 145
Papayas, shopping for, 186

Parkinson, James, 78
Parkinson's disease, 75, 78–79
  antioxidants and, 28
  free radicals and, 27–28, 79
  vitamin C and, 79, 80
  vitamin E and, 79–80
Parkinson Study Group, 80
Passwater, R. A., 139
Pastas
  easy vegetable primavera, 163
  gingered broccoli with pasta, 160–61
  red pepper spaghetti, 160
  vegetarian lasagna, 162
Pearl, Raymond, 24
Peas
  benefits of, 188
  shopping for, 188–89
Phenolic antioxidants, cancer and, 58
Physicians Health Study, 65, 67
Phytic acid, cancer and, 59
Phytochemicals, 5, 6, 8, 17, 109
  aging and, 5, 6, 11, 12, 18
  Alzheimer's disease and, 11, 18
  Antioxidant and Phytochemical
    advisory, 219–25
  arteriosclerosis and, 11, 18
  arthritis and, 11, 18
  benefits of, 56–57
  cancer and, 11, 18, 56–61
  cholesterol and, 16
  classes and compounds of, 219–25
  definition, 9
  diabetes and, 11, 18
  eye diseases and, 11, 18
  food sources of, 53, 57, 59–60, 185,
    187
  free radicals and, 10
  function of, 9, 10
  heart attack/stroke and, 11, 18
  hunter-gatherers and, 4–5
  osteoporosis and, 11, 18
  thymus and, 24
  see also Soy protein
Pierpaoli, W., 210
Pineal gland, 25
  as biological clock, 138, 204
  melatonin and, 138, 202, 207

Pintos, 189
Pizza
  red pepper, 158–59
  soy good, 159
Polyphenols
  cancer and, 58, 60, 61
  food sources of, 53, 129
Potter, J. D., 62
Precancerous cells, phytochemicals
  and, 58
Proanthocyanidins (PACs), Pycnogenol
  and, 139
Progression phase, of cancer, 59
Promotion phase, of cancer, 58
Prostaglandins, free radicals and, 27
Prostate cancer, 55, 208
  soy protein and, 12, 63, 109, 110,
    111, 116, 221
  see also Cancer
Protease inhibitors, cancer and, 59, 60
Pryor, William A., 7
Psyllium, in high-fiber diet, 100, 101
Pumpkin
  apricot pumpkin bread, 148
  pumpkin pie, 172
Purple grapes
  cancer and, 60, 61
  recommended daily intake of, 126
  shopping for, 186
Pycnogenol, 223–24
  recommended daily intake of, 126,
    139, 143, 213

R

Rate-of-living theory, see Metabolic
  theory of aging
Recipes
  for beverages, 170–71
  for breakfast, 144–51, 170
  for desserts, 146, 171–72
  for lunch/dinner, 152–69
  for snacks, 147–51, 169, 170–72
Red pepper pizza, 158–59
Red pepper spaghetti, 160
Red wine
  cancer and, 60, 61

Red wine (*cont.*)
  heart attack and, 46
  recommendations on, 141, 190, 215, 225
Regelson, W., 210
Reiter, Russel J., 201, 209, 210
Rest and relaxation, recommendations for, 127, 140, 215
Restaurant meals, recommendations for, 191
Rheumatoid arthritis, 91–92
  see also Arthritis
Richardson, J. Stephen, 28, 77
Richer, Stuart P., 102
Rimm, E. B., 42, 44
Robinson, Jo, 201
Running, benefits of, 178–79

S

Sahelian, Ray, 204
Salads
  citrus spinach, 152
  tomato-onion, 152
Seat belts, recommendations for, 127, 140, 215
Seddon, Johanna M., 103
Selenium, 52, 224
  cancer and, 54, 55, 62, 63, 68
Self-talk, motivation strengthened by, 195–96, 199
Sesame tofu stir-fry, 165–66
Shift workers, melatonin for, 204–5
Shopping, 184–90
  for beverages, 190
  for breads, cereals and crackers, 190
  for fruit, 185–87
  for soups, 189–90
  for vegetables, 187–89
Skin, 89–91
  antioxidants and, 90–91
  cancer of, 89, 90
  crow's feet, 89
  free radicals and, 89, 90
  function of, 89
  sunscreen and, 90–91
  ultraviolet (sun) damage to, 89, 90–91
  vitamin E and, 90, 91
  wrinkles, 89
Sleeping
  melatonin and, 201, 202–7, 210
  pills for, 141
  recommendations for, 140
Sloppy Joe surprise, 168
Smith, Charles D., 28
Smith, James R., 26
Smoking
  antioxidant, antiaging plan and, 126–27
  heart disease and, 48, 49
  supplements and, 64–65, 66, 68
  see also Nonsmoking
Snacks
  menu plans for, 133
  recipes for, 147–51, 169, 170–72
Snow peas, glazed snow peas and carrots, 157
Sodas, 190
Soups
  creamy spinach, 155
  curried carrot, 154
  gazpacho, 153–54
  shopping for, 189–90
  spicy tomato-onion, 155–56
Soybeans, 60, 61
Soy-good chocolate pudding, 171
Soy good pizza, 159
Soy milk, 190
Soy muffins, *see* Muffins
Soy protein, 107–22, 141
  aging and, 118
  cancer and, 12, 59, 63, 107–8, 109, 110, 111, 115–17, 121, 221
  cholesterol and, 12, 110, 111, 112–15, 117–18
  daidzein, 12, 60, 61, 110, 221, 222
  disease reversal and, 122
  estradiole compared to, 110–11, 117–18
  estrogen replacement and, 116, 118

Soy protein (*cont.*)
  food sources of, 53, 111, 118–120,
    121, 122, 130, *see also* Tofu
  general prevention and, 121
  genistein, 12, 59, 60, 61, 110–11,
    116, 221–22
  heart disease and, 12, 107–8, 112,
    114, 121, 221
  isoflavones and, 12, 17–18, 53,
    109–111, 112, 116, 117, 118, 120,
    see also daidzein; genistein,
    above
  monkey studies on, 114–15, 118
  osteoporosis and, 12, 107–8, 111,
    117
  recommended daily intake of, 111,
    113, 119–20, 121, 122, 126
  supplements, 12, 17–18, 120
  tailored protection and, 121
  tamoxifen compared to, 110–11,
    117–18
  worldwide importance of, 109
Spaghetti, *see* Pasta
Spicy tomato-onion soup, 155–56
Spinach
  citrus spinach salad, 152
  creamy spinach soup, 155
Spinal arthritis, *see* Ankylosing
    spondylitis
Stampfer, M. J., 42, 44
Steinmetz, K. A., 62
Stomach cancer, 58, 63
  see also Cancer
Strawberry-banana frosty, 170
Stress, heart disease and, 48, 49
Stroke, 35
  antioxidant, antiaging program and,
    34–40
  antioxidants and, 11, 18
  causes of, 36–40
  definition, 36
  diabetes and, 96
  garlic and, 221
  general prevention and, 51
  homocysteine and, 46
  phytochemicals and, 11, 18
  soy protein and, 12

  tailored protection and, 51–52
  see also Heart attack
Summer mixed greens, 158
Sun, skin damage from, 89, 90–91
Sunny fruit fiesta, 145–46
Sunscreens, 90–91
Super-easy your-choice muffins,
    151
Superoxide dimutase (SOD), arthritis
    and, 92–93
Supplements, 9, 12, 18, 127, 135–39,
    142, 215, 216–17
  aging and, 126
  amount of in diet, 52
  antioxidant, 127, 135–37, 142,
    213
  arguments against taking, 69
  aspirin, 51, 126, 138, 142, 213
  beta-carotene, 45, 52, 55
  brain function and, 85
  calcium, 136
  cancer and, 54–55, 63–69, 70, 71,
    126
  cataracts and, 104
  cholesterol and, 15, 16
  disease reversal and, 126, 127
  FABB, 126, 137, 213–14
  fish oil, 127, 137, 143, 213
  general prevention and, 126, 127,
    136–37
  heart disease and, 34, 35, 51, 52,
    126
  immune system and, 29–30
  iron, 136
  isoflavone, 120
  Pycnogenol, 126, 139, 143, 213
  recommended daily intake of, 127,
    142, 213–14
  selenium, 52, 54, 55, 224
  soy protein, 12, 17–18, 120
  tailored protection and, 126, 127
  vitamin C, 52, 219
  vitamin E, 52, 55, 219
  vitamin-mineral, 127, 136, 142, 213,
    219
  weight loss and, 13
  see also Melatonin

Sweet and sour tofu, 167
Swift, Jonathan, 87

T

Tacos, vegetarian, 165
Tailored protection, 18
  cancer and, 71
  diet and, 126
  exercise and, 126, 179, 181
  health-promoting habits and, 127
  heart disease/stroke and, 51–52
  lipids and, 47
  program for, 126–27
  soy protein and, 121
  supplements and, 126, 127, 137
Tamoxifen
  breast cancer and, 110–11, 117
  melatonin and, 208
  osteoporosis and, 117
  soy protein compared to, 110–11,
   117–18
Tangy vegetable juice, 171
Taste, calisthenics for sense of, 83
T cells, immune system and, 24
Tea, black, 141, 224–25
  see also Green tea
Thun, Michael, 67–68
Thymus, aging and, 23–24
Tocotrienols, cholesterol and, 109
Tofu, 72, 119, 121, 122
  sesame tofu stir-fry, 165–66
  sweet and sour, 167
  tofu sweet potato bake, 168–69
  vegetable tofu stir-fry, 166
  in vegetarian lasagna, 162
Tomato-onion salad, 153
Tomato-onion soup, spicy, 155–56
Touch, calisthenics for sense of, 83
Tranquilizers, 141
Triglycerides, 47
  antioxidant, antiaging program and,
   21, 32
  desirable levels of, 47–48
  fish oil and, 137
  test of, 51, 52
Tutti-fruitti, 170

Type I diabetes, 97
  see also Diabetes
Type II diabetes, 97–98, 99–100, 177
  see also Diabetes
Tyrosine kinase, genistein and, 59

U

Ultraviolet (UV) rays, skin damage
  from, 89, 90–91
Upper-body exercise, 126, 134–35,
  142, 173, 179–80, 181, 215–16
Uric acid, heart disease and, 48, 49

V

Vacations, recommendations on, 140,
  215
Van Der Hagen, Anita M., 104
Vegetable juice
  recommended daily intake of, 126
  tangy, 171
Vegetable medley, 157
Vegetables and fruits, 9, 12, 18,
  128–34, 141
  allium vegetables, 60, 129
  benefits of, 142
  beta-carotene and vitamin C content
   of, 129, 226–28
  cancer and, 60, 61–63, 68
  cruciferous vegetables, 60, 129
  fruit-ripening "bowl" and, 186
  honor roll of, 129
  recommended daily intake of, 126
  shopping for, 185–89
  worksheet for increasing intake of,
   130–31
Vegetable tofu stir-fry, 166
Vegetarian lasagna, 162
Vegetarian tacos, 165
Very-low-density lipoproteins
  (VLDLs), 37, 47
  see also Triglycerides
Viruses, free radicals and, 10
Visualization, motivation strengthened
  by, 196–98
Vitamin A, 6

Vitamin A (*cont.*)
  brain and, 78
  thymus and, 24
  see also Beta-carotene
Vitamin B$_6$, 46
  see also FABB supplement
Vitamin B$_{12}$, 46
  see also FABB supplement
Vitamin C, 6, 17
  amount of in diet, 52
  benefits of, 142
  brain and, 75, 78
  cancer and, 58, 59–60, 62, 63
  cataracts and, 103, 104
  cholesterol and, 16
  diabetes and, 99
  elderly deficient in, 29
  food sources of, 53, 185
  heart disease and, 34, 40, 42, 45
  Parkinson's disease and, 79, 80
  Pycnogenol and, 139
  recommendations on, 225
  recommended daily intake of, 127,
    136–37, 142, 219
  thymus and, 24
  vegetables and fruits containing,
    129, 226–28
  vitamin E and, 40, 45
  see also Antioxidants
Vitamin E, 5, 6, 17
  aging and, 26
  amount of in diet, 52
  arthritis and, 93
  benefits of, 142
  brain and, 75, 78
  cancer and, 54, 55, 58, 62, 63, 68
  cataracts and, 104
  cholesterol and, 16, 109
  diabetes and, 98, 99
  elderly deficient in, 29
  heart disease and, 29, 34, 40, 42, 43,
    44, 48, 49
  Parkinson's disease and, 79–80

  recommendations on, 225
  recommended daily intake of, 127,
    137, 142, 219
  for skin, 90, 91
  supplements, 52, 55, 219
  thymus and, 24
  vitamin C and, 40, 45
  see also Antioxidants
Vitamin-mineral supplements,
    recommended daily intake of,
    127, 136, 142, 213, 219
VLDLs, *see* Very-low-density
    lipoproteins

W

Walking, 126, 134, 135, 142, 173,
    178–80, 181–82, 183, 195–96,
    214
Wear-and-tear, free radical theory of
    aging, 26–28, 92
Weight loss/control
  diabetes and, 100
  diet and, 12–14, 17
  exercise and, 13, 14, 178, 179–80
White blood cells, free radicals and,
    10
Wilmore, Douglas W., 222–23
Wine, *see* Red wine
Workaholic, 141, 215
Wrinkles, 89
Wurtman, Richard J., 203–4

Y

Yolton, Diane P., 104
Yolton, Robert L., 104
Yoshikawa, Toshikazu, 79

Z

Zaridze, D., 63
Zinc, 225–26